T0198726

bOlder

Heart Health in the
Golden Years

Mohamed Shalaby, MD

BALBOA.PRESS
A DIVISION OF HAY HOUSE

Balboa Press books may be ordered through booksellers or by contacting:

Balboa Press
A Division of Hay House
1663 Liberty Drive
Bloomington, IN 47403
www.balboapress.com
844-682-1282

Print information available on the last page.

ISBN: 979-8-7652-3900-1 (sc)
ISBN: 979-8-7652-3899-8 (hc)
ISBN: 979-8-7652-3901-8 (e)

Library of Congress Control Number: 2023903340

Balboa Press rev. date: 02/15/2023

CONTENTS

♥

CHAPTER 1

THE MULTIPLE PATHS TO LONG AND HEALTHY LIFE

As we get older, it is only natural to be more concerned about one's health. As the physical body ages, bodily systems (like the cardiovascular system) which were once reliable to the point of being unremarkable, slowly begin to break down. Through their reduced ability, such systems make themselves known, and impossible to ignore. It thus becomes critical to form a body of knowledge with respect to health in old age, and how to maintain health. Such information is not necessarily useful in the treatment of common old age maladies -- because, of course, treatment is always best left to doctors, nurses, and other caregivers -- but *knowledge* can be critical to the prevention of age-related maladies, and to ensuring lasting health and happiness in one's golden years.

Imparting such knowledge is the purpose of this book.

What is health, anyway? Simply put, the concept of health refers to well-being, both of a physical and emotional sort. We can all remember what it feels like to be in good health. The lucky ones among us may even remember (or even continue to live their day-to-day lives) in strong emotional and mental health. Although health is thus a simpler concept than it might seem, it is also subjective, meaning that it varies from person to person. By extension, this subjectivity is the challenge of health care, where practitioners have the responsibility to help each of their unique patients to achieve states of optimal health.

It is this idea of *optimal* health which guides the current discussion, and informs much of the work to follow. For the individuals older than age 65 who form the central 'audience' for this book, it is likely an understandable but forgone conclusion that they will not be able to return to the feeling of health and vitality of their youth. Sadly, while this is true, health and happiness can be maintained in old age. In fact, the task of old age is to ensure that *quality of life* is maintained, especially through **retaining functional mobility, awareness, and limiting pain.** While old age can be a time of lesser vitality, there is no reason why the elderly cannot live lives of dignity and satisfaction, pursue their interests with vigor, and have pleasurable, enjoyable days.

Some readers may believe that it is less the responsibility of the individual to look after their own health, as that of doctors and nurses and other healthcare professionals. Although this is certainly the case when it comes to emergency and even routine care, the best means by which optimal health outcomes can be achieved is through continual *preventive health behaviors.* While such health behaviors can, and often must be taught by licensed care professionals, it remains the responsibility of the individual to look after their own day-to-day health. This book intends to present facts and recommendations to help guide such self care.

Additionally, this personal responsibility for maintaining one's own health is particularly acute in the United States. While the U.S. has some of the world's highest health expenditures, this has not necessarily resulted in superior health outcomes for the American population. In 2017, according to data released by the Centers for Disease Control and Prevention (CDC), healthcare costs in the United States were $3.5 trillion. Despite this huge cost, Americans have lower life expectancy and frequently poorer quality of life than people in other developed countries. Unsurprisingly, such negative outcomes disproportionately fall upon the elderly, that is, Americans over age 65. Notably, while the American health system is replete with waste and inefficiency, the American lifestyle is also unhealthy. Poor lifestyle choices like smoking and sedentary living contribute to many of these poor health outcomes over time.

It is not difficult to recognize the potential for lifestyle and behavioral changes to cause notable improvements in long-term health outcomes; when combined with a healthy and active role in medical care, it is reasonable to argue that elderly individuals are the strongest **stewards** of their health.

The sort of stewardship that we're talking about here is more commonly known as *preventive care*. It consists of habits and behaviors taken as a precaution, with full knowledge of the scientific data and expert recommendations, and with the goal of living a long and healthy life. Unfortunately, this is not a simple task. As noted by Spalding (2008), preventive healthcare decision making and associated recommendations increase in complexity over the lifespan. This is understandable, given the huge complexity of body systems, especially as they begin to break down.

A promising place to start making such recommendations concerns the **leading causes of death**. Although it may seem a bit morbid to consider, the elderly patient (and the reader of this volume) is ultimately looking to optimize their quality of life and improve their lifespan, and effectively, to fight against death itself. To this end, here they are: The leading causes of death in the U.S. are malignant neoplasm (cancer), cerebral vascular disease, chronic lower respiratory disease, and heart disease. Many of these mortality outcomes are tightly associated with leading behavioral causes of death, including physical inactivity, tobacco use (smoking and chewable), and poor diet, especially consisting of food which is high in sugar or trans fats.

In the broadest sense, preventative care for individuals older than age 65 is recommended to focus upon quitting smoking and improving diet, as well as regimens of aerobic exercise and strength training. Adults in this age bracket should also focus upon preventive care through vaccinations, including those against tetanus, diphtheria, pneumococcal infection, and influenza. Aspirin therapy and lipid management is also recommended. What is the 'take-away' here? **The health of the individual over age 65 must be considered 'global' in nature**, meaning that all of the systems of the body, as well as behavior, outlook, and psychology must be optimized to achieve effective outcomes. Once again, by 'effective' outcomes, we mean happiness and long life.

One physical aspect of the body critical to this consideration is **heart health**. Although there are multiple major organs who's smooth running is necessary for health and well-being, none are as crucial to life as the heart. As will be considered in strong detail throughout this book, heart health is of critical importance, both with respect to the patient-physician relationship, and the responsibility which the individual has to look after their own health. Indeed, preventive behaviors and actions which focus upon heart health are the most beneficial to long-term positive health outcomes.

But what of other aspects of health? This book places great emphasis upon means by which physical health, and especially heart health can be optimized in old age. However, without the more complex state of **psychological fulfillment**, even a heart-healthy old age can be marred by depression or other mental health disorders.

As an effective means of encapsulating the concept of psychological fulfillment, it is important to consider the *hierarchy of needs* advanced by Abraham Maslow (1943). The author proposed that the 'base' of this hierarchy (those most central to survival) consists of physical needs, such as food and shelter. More advanced needs -- supported by the achievement of lower-order needs -- include social esteem, success in work or at home, and ultimately, self-fulfillment (or 'self-actualization'). This final goal of self-actualization is strongly linked to happiness, and is essentially the strongest personal achievement to which anyone can aspire. Like health in the physical body, achieving fulfillment in one's mind and outlook is complex, difficult to achieve, and subjective in nature. There is a galaxy of different paths that can be taken toward meeting this important goal.

Unfortunately, adults whose lives have been marked by poor emotional support are likelier to manifest with maladaptive coping mechanisms, and are poorly-positioned to achieve psychological fulfillment. Instead, they are likely to manifest any number of mental health disorders. The consequences of such disorders may be ruinous to physical health as well, due to poor mental health so often going hand in hand with neglect for physical care and substance abuse. As a result, the goal of social and psychological fulfillment is best considered as important as goals prioritizing care for one's physical health. Notably, **superior social support, as well as the presence of caring loved ones**, lead to superior health outcomes due to social responsibility. Put simply, the more people who care about you, the better, because there are more people who can look after you, but also because you have more people to live for.

A closely associated principle most commonly associated with achieving health for long life is economic stability, also known as 'peace of mind'. This book will consider that concept in stronger detail in a later chapter. However, simply, economic stability and freedom from poverty and deprivation are associated with a longer and healthier life. Individuals older than age 65 are eligible for Medicare in the United States, as well as for Social Security, both of which facilitate the elderly person's ability to avoid common pitfalls of old age in the past. That said, access to subsidized healthcare and a monthly stipend from the government are not necessarily enough to achieve the peace of mind upon which mental health and indeed, physical wellness, will often depend. Instead, it is often in the best interests of elderly individuals to maintain and even cultivate interests and hobbies, especially when such interests are stimulating and can contribute to a robust financial income. This might seem like a suggestion to continue working a job. But if not leisure, what is the purpose of retirement? However, as this book will show, conventional retirement -- meaning the cessation of work and employment -- may be not as beneficial as it appears during a strenuous working career. In fact, multiple benefits may be appreciated from continuing to work, especially in a job which you enjoy.

First, continuing to work means continuing to earn income. Although Social Security money and Medicare health insurance provide a robust 'safety net', individuals older than age 65 may find that living off of such benefits alone is insufficient to maintain the lifestyle they developed while working full-time. The result is that while the temptation runs strong to stop working all together and enjoy one's retirement, the capacity for enjoyment in such retirement is lower when quality of life is reduced. This may lead to negative mental health outcomes which ultimately endanger physical health.

One promising alternative is to find, or to maintain, employment which is stimulating for otherwise fulfilling. This can provide a useful degree of supplemental income as well. However, it is the element of fulfillment which is most crucial to recommendations to continue to work after the 'retirement' age. Economic stability and peace of mind are chief among the benefits of taking this path.

However, the core principle embodied by this proposal is the idea that health in long life, and in particular, psychological fulfillment in old age, can result in a feeling of *usefulness*. Much evidence indicates that people have an intrinsic need to be useful to others. As social beings, humans do not lose this need in old age, despite norms which support the idea that retirement should be spent in idle relaxation. To this end, mental health and financial peace of mind may both be served through continuing to work, particularly at a job which one finds fulfilling. Additionally, the fulfillment of the need to feel useful may also be achieved through contributing to housework, child care, and volunteer work, depending on the needs and abilities of the person or family in question.

It might be hard to believe, but scientific as well as anecdotal evidence supports the usefulness of continuing to work even during your 'retirement' years. In fact, you might know someone in your own life who retired from work and then, seemingly for no reason, passed away shortly thereafter. This is not a coincidence. Although all-cause mortality rates among retirees is higher among individuals with lower income and education, the general findings of multiple studies supports the idea that once people no longer have a 'reason' to live -- as grave as that may seem -- their life expectancy drops precipitously. In particular, individuals whose identity as fulfilled and even defined by work during their career tend to find it very difficult to adapt to the new realities of retirement life.

Individuals who retire from work altogether may come to feel lost, unsure of who they are and how they should be spending their time. As a result, they become particularly susceptible to inactivity, both of a physical and mental sort, and are more likely to present with physical problems flowing from sedentary lifestyle, or mental illness. In some cases, the unexpected crisis of identity which follows full retirement from work may result in mental health consequences such as depression, as well as the potential for associated negative behavioral consequences such as alcohol or substance abuse. Additionally, the negative consequences which result from difficulty in achieving personal fulfillment in old age may result in other problem behaviors considered in this chapter. Overeating, for instance, or eating unhealthy foods, is often the result of maladaptive coping, and can result in damage to the heart and other vital organs.

It is in this context that this discussion returns to the heart, the health of which forms the central 'core' of the work and recommendations to follow. Put simply, the mental and physical health needs of old age are wide reaching in nature, and are reflected in not merely the physical body but the mind and the social experience of being human. If one or more of these critical areas of concern is neglected, as by insufficient or inadequate medical care, poor community contacts, or behaviors, or an unhealthy psychological outlook, the heart is often the first organ to suffer. Because the heart is so crucial to life, it is important to remember the wide range of ways in which various behaviors contribute to or detract from heart health. That assessment will form the basis for the chapters to follow.

This book aims to provide a working guide for healthy living in old age, with a focus upon the heart, but also a wide range of other factors from which overall physical health is the result. Mental health will be placed under the umbrella of physical health, insofar as the mind is situated within the brain, maintaining healthful living requires psychological health. Once again, however, the heart -- and the health thereof -- will form the central focus of this overview, with additional topics related back to this focus.

Chapters to follow will evaluate a range of topics. **Chapter 2, Health Throughout The Life Cycle** will evaluate health throughout the life cycle, as a means of establishing a foundation for recognizing the ways in which elderly healthcare can be optimized. It will consider adaptive and not adaptive factors during different phases of the life cycle, and offer a review of this complex topic. **Chapter 3, Preventive Care Overview** will expand upon the present consideration of preventive care and the criticality of preventive care in the elderly. The prevention of cardiovascular disease and in particular, means of achieving optimal heart health will be emphasized. Cancer screening, major comorbidities, and healthcare engagement will all be evaluated in strong detail, leaving into major recommendations for healthcare practice and priorities for elderly readers. **Chapter 4, Heart Anatomy and Change Over the Lifespan** will build upon some of the lifespan factors evaluated in chapter 2, but with particular concern paid to the effects of old age on heart health, and the particular cardiovascular risk factors which are experienced by elderly individuals. This, too, will flow into specific recommendations for the elderly reader. Chapter 5, **Modifiable Risk Factors for Atherosclerosis,** will consider the particular lifestyle changes which are necessary in order to improve heart health outlook over time. This will include an overview of smoking and tobacco use cessation, as well as the risk factors for poor heart health posed by psychosocial stressors, lack of exercise, and overall sedentary lifestyle. Additionally, hypocholesterolemia and other particular heart specific risk factors will be considered for their prevalence and the relative risk factor they pose to elderly individuals. **Chapter 6, Optimizing Heart Health in Old Age,** will consider both common medications which are used to help maintain the health of the heart and cardiovascular system, as well as habits and lifestyle choices which may also achieve the same goals. **Chapter 7, Mental Health and Stress and Heart Health in Old Age,** will evaluate the mental health risks which result in heart disease or stroke, especially the phenomenon of stress resulting in acute risks to cardiovascular health. Evidence will be considered to link the problem of stress to the reduced physical resilience or incapacity to maintain bodily homeostasis, which often comes from old age. Stress related cardiac inflammation will also be considered, particularly for its potential to result in late life depression and other mental illness. **Chapter 8, Reducing Stress and Optimizing Psychological Fulfillment**, will contain a wide variety of recommendations upon which optimal Health outcomes, particularly related to the heart, can be achieved. This chapter will consider recommendations for physical exercise in elderly adults, as well as particular strategies by which mental health and old age can be optimized. Mental health will be distinguished from psychological health; insofar as mental disorders pose a greater threat to heart health outcomes than poor relationships or an ill-defined identity. The importance of continuing work, or at least maintaining a sense of purpose, will be highlighted as crucial to achieving psychological fulfillment. **Chapter 9, Productivity and Peace of Mind in Old Age**, will continue this evaluation of ways in which stress outcomes most associated with poor cardiovascular health can be reduced. Financial instability and peace of mind will be considered in greater detail. Primary recommendations flowing from this chapter will emphasize minimizing stress, either from financial factors or the threat of scarcity. Finally, **Chapter**

10, Overview and Overall Recommendations, will present a range of recommendations, both specific and general, flowing from the discussions in the prior chapters. In particular, such recommendations will center upon physical health in general, heart health in particular, reducing stress related heart health risks, maintaining mental health, and finally, the importance of identity and goal setting.

REFERENCES

Centers for Disease Control and Prevention (2021). *Health Expenditures.* Retrieved from https://www.cdc.gov/nchs/fastats/health-expenditures.htm

Haraldstad, K., Wahl, A., Andenæs, R., Andersen, J. R., Andersen, M. H., Beisland, E., ... & Helseth, S. (2019). A systematic review of quality of life research in medicine and health sciences. *Quality of life Research, 28*(10), 2641-2650.

Kim, J., Kim, J., Kim, Y., Han, A., & Nguyen, M. C. (2021). The contribution of physical and social activity participation to social support and happiness among people with physical disabilities. *Disability and Health Journal, 14*(1), 100974.

Maslow, A. H. (1943). A theory of human motivation. *Psychological review, 50*(4), 370.

Picchio, M., & van Ours, J. C. (2020). Mental health effects of retirement. *De Economist, 168*(3), 419-452.

Reimann, Z., Miller, J. R., Dahle, K. M., Hooper, A. P., Young, A. M., Goates, M. C., ... & Crandall, A. (2020). Executive functions and health behaviors associated with the leading causes of death in the United States: A systematic review. *Journal of health psychology, 25*(2), 186-196.

Spalding, M. C., & Sebesta, S. C. (2008). Geriatric screening and preventive care. *American family physician, 78*(2), 206-216.

Tóth-Király, I., Bőthe, B., Orosz, G., & Rigó, A. (2020). On the importance of balanced\need fulfillment: A person-centered perspective. *Journal of Happiness Studies*, *21*(6), 1923-1944.

Urbich, M., Globe, G., Pantiri, K., Heisen, M., Bennison, C., Wirtz, H. S., & Di Tanna, G. L.(2020). A systematic review of medical costs associated with heart failure in the USA (2014–2020). *PharmacoEconomics*, 1-18.

♥

CHAPTER 2

HEALTH THROUGHOUT THE LIFE CYCLE

NOW THAT WE HAVE DELVED into the larger themes that will inform this work as a whole, it is necessary to evaluate means by which overall health -- and especially, *heart* health -- can be improved and optimized throughout the life cycle. The life cycle is a concept with which many readers may no doubt consider themselves familiar. It begins with infancy and childhood, and progresses through adulthood and old age, and ends, inevitably, in death. Where many might not have as strong a body of knowledge is with respect to how health can be optimized during the different phases of life. Still fewer may understand the differences between stages of life where one is actually able to take measures to ensure and protect their health, and stages in which one is essentially, 'not in control'. The prospect of being out of control, or otherwise being unable to improve or even sustain one's health may result in the reader feeling depressed or confused. However, I am here to say that the vast majority of the lifespan allows the individual to exercise a great deal of control over their 'health destiny', so to speak. What remains are the periods of life when the individual is dependent or otherwise requires the help of others, be they friends, family, or medical professionals, to sustain their good health. It is thus the responsibility of the individual to maintain their good health when they are able, so as to not exert too great a burden upon family or caregivers during phases of life when they cannot care for themselves. Of course, quality of life certainly plays a role in making these determinations, but I have found most of my patients prefer to not exert too great a burden upon their family and caregivers, no matter their age or capacity. For this reason, I have found that most of my patients are receptive to the idea of caring for themselves when they have the mental and physical capacity to do so. Again, in order to understand the different degrees of responsibility which the individual has to maintain their own health, it is crucial to recognize the differences between the stages of the *life cycle*. An evaluation of these stages follows below:

THE LIFE CYCLE

In the broadest sense, it is perhaps common knowledge that different stages of life have different degrees of relevance and even importance to health outcomes. To this end, it is useful to employ a **life course** approach to health, and the optimization thereof, particularly with respect to heart health. As considered in chapter 1, health can be defined as a state of well-being which extends not only to one's physical body, but to mental and social outcomes as well. The goal of health throughout the lifespan, but particularly during certain stages, is to reduce mortality and morbidity. One must also reduce the particular determinants of poor health, such as behavioral and environmental factors. Smoking, in particular, offers a key example of a behavioral factor with a negative impact upon health. Although it is certainly possible for an individual to smoke for many decades without serious -- that is, recognizable -- health consequences, the tragedy of the life course approach to health is that by the time the smoker begins to feel the consequences of this deadly habit, it is often too late for them to do anything about it.

It is because of examples such as smoking that the life course approach to health is generally grouped into **adaptive** (controllable) and **non-adaptive** (uncontrollable) features of different phases of the human life cycle. Once again, this may come across as a somewhat painful revelation, but there are phases of the life cycle where, put simply, one's health is not in their own hands. It is not difficult to recognize that the period from childbirth through infancy, childhood, and adolescence represents one such time. However, lesser known is the way in which health problems and challenges accrued over the course of adulthood contribute to a similar **lack of health agency** between the years 60 and 90, and especially after age 90. It may seem a foregone conclusion that one must take better care of their health after age 60, and certainly after age 90. However, it is crucial to recognize that the purpose of healthcare during those ages is to *maintain* health, that is, to work under the health (and well-being) 'ceiling' fostered due to behavioral, environmental, and physical traits and characteristics adopted or avoided during the adaptive phases of the life cycle.

Beginning with **early life**, the years between birth and age 20 can result in a wide range of health outcomes based upon factors which are not necessarily in the control of the young individual. These can include genetic factors, differential socioeconomic status, and differential educational outcomes, all of which contribute to superior or inferior health results both during those years and in later life.

The adaptive phases of the life cycle are those times in life when the individual has the capacity, energy, and will to exercise control over their own health maintenance and health-related behavioral practice. These are generally the years between ages 20 and 50, as well as the transitional years between age 50 and 65. During those **formative and transitional years**, it is possible to focus on optimizing educational attainment, healthy habits, physical activity, and other factors which contribute to long-term health and wellness. During the **transitional years** (ages 50 to 65), the adaptive health related factors to be optimized include family relationships, career attainment, and general lifestyle factors. If properly attended to, these can result in maintenance of beneficial health habits.

Finally, after age 65, and especially after age 90, the individual is increasingly less able to take care of their own health. As a result, **the elderly years** witness an increasing number of non-adaptive factors determining longevity, but also a host of adaptive factors such as family, companionship, passions and interests, physical security, and finally that of general Health and well-being. Put simply, after age 65, it is crucial for the individual to receive strong and effective health care, but -- as considered in Chapter 1 -- longevity is also partially dependent on the individual having a *reason* to go on living. The existence of passions and interests is thus crucial for the elderly individual. In short, overall health is largely dependent upon upbringing and health maintenance during formative early childhood years, but longevity requires that environmental and behavioral factors are attended to during adaptive phases of the life cycle (that is, in adulthood). Finally, living to old age requires a combination of adaptive and non-adaptive factors, particularly access to effective health care, the presence of passions and other personal interests, and access to supportive family and friends.

MORTALITY AND NON-ADAPTIVE FACTORS

Before this work considers the central factors most strongly connected to longevity, it is crucial to point out that mortality rates in the United States reached all-time lows in 2019. Life expectancy at birth, appropriately, attained record highs during that year, reaching 81.1 years for women and 76.1 years for men, leading to an overall average life expectancy of roughly 78.5 years. Important context for these figures can be taken from the life expectancy at birth for Americans born in the year 1960. That year, the life expectancy for American women was a mere 73.1 years, while men's life expectancy was only 66.6 years. The past 50 years have thus seen an increase in life expectancy of 8 years for women and nearly a decade for men. These figures should provide the reader with some confidence and understanding of the advances that have been made over the last 50 years, particularly with respect to long-term elderly and even end of life care. Put simply, more Americans have greater access to more effective health care. Unfortunately, what these figures do not indicate is the host of non-adaptive -- that is environment-focused and social -- factors which have grown alongside these overall trends in longevity improvement and decreasing trends in all-cause mortality.

When it comes to factors that influence health but which are not always recognized as such, first and foremost is **socioeconomic status.** This is a more complicated concept than simple income or wealth, and takes into account social standing and privilege as well. Generally, SES flows from measures of financial security. Perhaps unsurprisingly, there is a strong link between socioeconomic status and life expectancy. One study from Canada (Bilal et al., 2019) showed that there were significant health disparities between individuals of low and high socioeconomic status, even when accounting for the Canadian social safety net and in particular, the universal health care in that nation. Like most developed nations the world over, Canadian citizens are entitled to health coverage funded through direct taxation. Researchers used a wide ranging sample of over 6 million subjects to find, shockingly, that Canadian men and women in the lowest socioeconomic status group live an average of 12 and 9 years less than men and women in the higher socioeconomic status (SES) group.

Let's consider that again: Even in Canada, a country with universal healthcare, it would appear that 'money talks', and that individuals with higher income, net worth, and social privilege are better-able to afford or access the services which allow them to live longer lives. Results of this Canadian study indicated that the link between SES and health outcomes appears to be a universal phenomenon, but is present even in a nation where social policy is designed to engender health equity. In addition, these researchers found that the lower the SES, the higher the odds of death, independent of age.

By extension, it can be recognized that in the United States -- the only nation in the developed (wealthy) world which does not provide universal health care -- there is an even stronger connection between wealth/SES and longevity. It can thus be argued that in the US, health outcomes are even more skewed (than Canada) to favor those of higher wealth, income, or SES. Putting it simply, not only do the wealthy live longer lives, **but it is essentially unhealthy to be poor.** Stepping away from any assessment of comparative social policy across Western nations, this finding seems to indicate that wealth, income, and SES are each closely linked to health outcomes generally outside of the control of the individual. Moreover, the wealthy are effectively 'freed' to engage in certain high-risk behaviors, confident in their ability to receive effective treatment if and when they suffer adverse consequences. A central example of this phenomenon regards the choice to take certain drugs of abuse, or compulsive behaviors in general. While the wealthy are just as likely to develop addiction or compulsive behaviors, they are more likely to receive effective treatment, and for this reason, behavioral or environmental health stressors pose less of a direct health threat. By contrast, poor people -- individuals of low SES -- must make consistently appropriate health decisions, because treatment in the event of addiction, illness or injury can carry insurmountable costs. The end result of these phenomena is that wealth, income, and SES also tends to influence the likelihood of individuals to live into extreme old age. Another study, (Lailo & Raitano, 2018) explored life expectancy in old age and found life expectancy at age 60 to differ by five years across subjects of low and high SES, with the higher life expectancy outcomes among subjects whose financial situation was more secure.

Another generally not adaptive factor which is also closely related to longevity is **educational attainment**. One study (Hummer et al., 2013) found that American citizens who are more highly educated live longer lives, on average. This study found that educational attainment serves as a fundamental cause of health and life expectancy. However, there is some question as to the degree to which educational attainment 'follows' SES. In other words, it is not unreasonable to predict that individuals with longer lifespans are the same individuals able to afford high educational attainment. It might thus be indicated that higher levels of educational attainment do not necessarily cause people to live long lives, but those with such attainment tend to live longer.

In total, a wide range of non-adaptive factors contribute to overall health and longevity outcomes. Notably, while the overall lifespan and life expectancy in the United States has increased considerably over the last 50 years, so has income and wealth inequality. This means that to the extent that SES determines health outcomes, such health outcomes are becoming more and more unequal, and with them the environmental or behavioral health risks faced by the majority of the US population. Unfortunately, SES factors prominently in the ability of individuals to obtain and afford critical preventive care. This can mean that for individuals in life stages where they can 'adapt' to health challenges, most are not playing on an even playing field, even in nations with universal healthcare or equitable access to education. The result is that low SES is a heart health -- and overall health -- risk in itself.

ACTIVITY, RESILIENCE AND SOCIALIZATION

Given this chapter's indication that socioeconomic status (SES) and educational status are strong correlates of long life, the reader may be curious which behaviors constitute **appropriately adaptive traits during the lifespan**. One means by which long life may be better assured is through **exercise and physical activity**, with multiple studies indicating the relationship between physical activity and increased lifespan. This is a critical recommendation given the close connection between physical activity and increased heart strength and heart health with respect to reducing the threat of adverse heart related incidents such as stroke or infarction. Daily exercise, in particular, or exercise which is incorporated into daily life, has been shown to have a stronger impact on lifespan then other factors. Notably, exercise -- particularly cardiovascular exercise such as jogging or bicycling -- is associated with stronger heart health and lifespan, and these are relatively simple and inexpensive habits to adopt. This is why I believe that the most important recommendation that I can provide to my patients is to **begin exercising and enjoying exercise, earlier in life**. Although it is not impossible to adopt a cardiovascular exercise regimen after the age of 60, it can be very difficult to do so. Much of the same recommendations can be made for proper diet, with the formative years of the life cycle (ages 20 to 50) also those in which the individual has the greatest capacity to engage in health-adaptive diet behaviors most conducive to long life.

Another behavior and health related trait which is somewhat adaptive and which is critical to long life is known as **resiliency**. This concept is born out of research that aimed to determine why elderly individuals, despite their multiple health problems and increasing infirmity, also tend to present with lower levels of psychopathology when compared to the general population. The prevailing understanding of this phenomenon points to resiliency, a characteristic of individuals who have overcome adversity. They increasingly do not worry about the challenges ahead because of the many challenges they have overcome. Resiliency is a trait developed over a lifetime, but which is said to 'fully flower' in old age. Resiliency is a capacity to overcome challenges and to maintain one's health and function despite loss, disability, or disease. The phenomenon of 'resilience thinking', in particular, is linked to superior health outcomes as well as a stronger sense of personal well-being and peace of mind.

In order to achieve resiliency thinking, our recommendations again return to the general purpose of longevity, namely to continue the pursuit of one's passions and interests. Individuals who have a strong purpose in life, be it connection to family, their career, or their personal interests and hobbies, are more likely to be able to rebound from adversity. Resilience becomes a means to an end, and as such represents a significant adaptive trait which can help to ensure health and well-being into old age.

Finally, it is necessary to touch upon the importance of **friendships, family, and general companionship** as a boon to heart health, alongside general health and longevity. Social relationships are adaptive and crucial for survival, meaning that direct correlations can be drawn between the number and strength of social relationships and the capacity of individuals to maintain their health and long life. A contrasting example is drawn from the host of studies which have shown that social isolation -- as considered in Chapter 1 -- is linked to poor health.

It is thus crucial for individuals to engage in healthy relationships and to maintain them throughout the lifespan, to achieve a host of beneficial outcomes. Personal friendships and companionship have been shown, in particular, to improve immune response, to release hormones which reduce stress, to improve digestion, to better regulate blood sugar, and to improve self-esteem. Most notably for the purposes of this work, friendships have been shown to improve cardiovascular health and longevity.

DISCUSSION

Health and happiness throughout the lifespan is often a matter of personal choices, but it can also depend upon a host of genetic, environmental, and socioeconomic factors over which the individual has little to no control. As a result, it is crucial for anyone interested in heart health and long life to recognize the 'hand they've been dealt', so to speak. While wealth and financial security can lead to improved long-term outcomes, they also provide a stronger 'safety net' against the consequences of negative health behaviors. Unfortunately, for the majority of readers without high SES, it is crucial to make health decisions which recognize their financial situation. Education, too, is another determinant of mortality and longevity, but for individuals for whom expensive education is not feasible, recommendations center upon informed personal health decisions. Such decisions can center upon heart healthy behaviors, particularly cardiovascular exercise and healthy diet. Moreover, making and maintaining lasting friendships and family bonds is also shown to improve overall long-term health. In short, in the absence of wealth, one must be wise, and wisdom means engaging in beneficial, heart-healthy behaviors to the greatest extent that one is able.

REFERENCES

Bilal, U., Cainzos-Achirica, M., Cleries, M., Santaeugènia, S., Corbella, X., Comin-Colet, J., & Vela, E. (2019). Socioeconomic status, life expectancy and mortality in a universal healthcare setting: An individual-level analysis of> 6 million Catalan residents. *Preventive Medicine, 123,* 91-94.

Busschbach, J. J., Hessing, D. J., & De Charro, F. T. (1993). The utility of health at different stages in life: a quantitative approach. Social Science & Medicine, 37(2), 153-158.

Carey, J. R. (2003). *Longevity: the biology and demography of life span.* Princeton University Press.

Edwards, K. A., Alschuler, K. A., Ehde, D. M., Battalio, S. L., & Jensen, M. P. (2017). Changes in resilience predict function in adults with physical disabilities: a longitudinal study. *Archives of physical medicine and rehabilitation, 98*(2), 329-336.

Harvard Health Publishing (2010). *The health benefits of strong relationships.* Retrieved from https://www.health.harvard.edu/staying-healthy/the-health-benefits-of-strong-relationships

Hummer, R. A., & Hernandez, E. M. (2013). The effect of educational attainment on adult mortality in the United States. *Population bulletin*, *68*(1), 1.

Holt-Lunstad, J. (2018). Why social relationships are important for physical health: A systems approach to understanding and modifying risk and protection. *Annual review of psychology*, *69*, 437-458.

Holt-Lunstad, J., Smith, T. B., & Layton, J. B. (2010). Social relationships and mortality risk: a meta-analytic review. *PLoS medicine*, *7*(7), e1000316.

Kennedy, H. L. (2021). *Aging and Health for the US Elderly: A Health Primer for Ages 60 to 90 Years*. University of Missouri Press.

Lallo, C., & Raitano, M. (2018). Life expectancy inequalities in the elderly by socioeconomic status: evidence from Italy. *Population health metrics*, *16*(1), 1-21.

Simply Insurance (2022). *Average US Life Expectancy Statistics by Gender, Ethnicity, State*. Retrieved from https://www.simplyinsurance.com/average-us-life-expectancy-statistics/#:~:text=Male%3A%2076.1%20years%20%2D%20Average%20life,US%20female%20(at%20birth).

CHAPTER 3

♥

PREVENTIVE CARE OVERVIEW

O NE OF THE MOST IMPORTANT lessons I've have taken from my years as a caregiver regards the importance of preventive care. It is never enough to begin from the point of crisis, particularly a life-threatening one such as a stroke or heart attack, and to use that crisis as a 'wake up call' to begin paying close attention to your health. Instead, it is crucial to consider your family history of adverse health events, and the statistical likelihoods and probabilities regarding which afflictions are likeliest to affect you. None of us can look forward to a life utterly free of adverse health events. At the same time, none of us is free of the specter of death. As much as it may pain us to consider, these facts mean that it is crucial to consider your life past age 50 as a series of **statistical probabilities** that would ideally be used to determine one's preventative health outlook.

What do I mean by this recommendation to use statistical probability to inform your preventive care outlook? It's simple.

There are simply not enough hours in the day to devote your full and uninterrupted attention to the different potential health threats that may arise. Instead, there are statistical likelihoods and best practices which you can use soberly in order to inform a focused and understanding health posture, one which is tailored to your needs. Too great a degree of concern regarding different health threats can result in paranoia, diminished quality of life, and most critically, may distract from obtaining the preventive care you need, that is, care tailored to the adverse events most likely to happen to you over age 50. It is crucial to begin to consider your life as composed of different potential adverse health events. Past age 50, the rate and severity of such adverse events goes up precipitously, but some events remain far more likely to occur than others.

Again, while this may seem obvious, I have found that many people are either unwilling or incapable of recognizing the different statistical probabilities defining adverse health events to which they are exposed as a factor of heredity, environment or behavior. It is for this reason that the necessity of confronting the health dangers of latter middle age and old age with a keen eye is so critical. If you take one lesson from this chapter, let it be this: **you can't prepare for everything, so you must prepare for the health threats which are more likely to affect you.**

One important place to start evaluating the different potential health risks of later middle age (past age 50) regards taking steps to prevent or forestall the known leading causes of death. This is a better place to begin because the 'short list' regarding leading causes of death is orders of magnitude less extensive than the number of potential health concerns which do not immediately cause or otherwise lead to mortality.

I think we would all agree that the most important goal of healthcare and especially prevention is the prevention of death itself, meaning that to confront the known leading causes of death represents an optimal prevention standpoint. In light of these concept, let's consider those leading causes of death in the United States:

Cancer. Described by some as the 'Emperor of Maladies', cancer is not one specific condition, but rather an 'umbrella' term to describe a certain dysfunctional state which afflicts the cells of the body. Cancer occurs when cells do not die at the normal point during their life cycle, and the unchecked growth of such cells begins to interfere with important or even essential, life maintaining body systems. In the United States, nearly 600,000 deaths from cancer occurred in 2017, meaning that cancer accounted for 21.3% of total deaths during that year (CDC, 2022b).

Cancer is one of the most devastating of all illnesses, but not in every case. Indeed, cancer is notable for its sheer variety, with some types – like skin cancer – often not only visible with the naked eye but perfectly capable of being removed (i.e. cured) with simple surgery. Other forms of cancer can be especially insidious, with the malignant sorts of lymphatic and pancreatic cancers, in particular, having a close to 100% mortality rate (CDC, 2022b). Familial history and behavioral factors certainly play a strong role in determining whether or not cancer presents as a threat. Additionally, exposure to environmental carcinogens varies widely across the population, with some groups having far higher cancer risk as a result of such environmental factors and others being relatively unaffected. However, it is important that the reader not 'waste their time' with excess worry about cancer mortality. What do I mean by this? It's perhaps old news, and I hope that the reader excuses this diversion, but there are **few comprehensive or effective preventive health measures that can be taken** to 'prevent' cancer, at least, not in the way that we currently understand 'prevention.'

In the face of such a complex and diverse grouping of bodily malady as cancer, it is perhaps more appropriate to focus upon behavioral and lifestyle changes that have been associated with a reduced cancer risk, but there are no 'cure-all' options or 'magic bullet' solutions to eliminating risk of cancer outright. Even when individuals abstain from behaviors known to cause malignant cancer – quitting smoking, for instance – a non-zero risk of cancer remains. Let's consider those statistics for a moment: Quitting smoking (as opposed to continuing to smoke) results in a 30% to 50% reduction in lung cancer risk over 10 years. However, this indicates that overall lung cancer risk remains 50-70% among even those smokers who quit (Taylor et al., 2002). Conversely, cancer of the mouth or esophagus is cut in half by quitting, so this behavior intervention results in a 50-50 risk of mouth or esophageal cancer even after quitting smoking (Taylor et al., 2002). However, because cancer reflects an error in replication at the very cellular level, it is perhaps best considered something of a 'natural disaster,' perhaps akin to being struck by lightning. Considered in this way, it is perhaps more appropriate to concern oneself about natural disasters local to your area – floods or tornadoes, for instance – then it is to concern oneself about cancer. Now of course, please do not take this review of probability as any sort of endorsement of negative health behaviors such as smoking. Instead, the intention of this section has been to touch upon the idea that out of all of the illnesses that can be fully prevented through behavioral or lifestyle changes past age 50, it is wise to not consider cancer one of them.

Other Causes of Death. Cancer may be one of the best known causes of death, but it is also something of an 'outlier' with respect to the possibilities available before the modern individual over age 50, with respect to optimizing their health outlook moving forward. Other leading causes of death include (1) *Cerebrovascular disease.* This is something of a catch-all term for the wide array of medical conditions that affect and afflict the blood vessels of the brain as well as blood circulation within the brain. The most typical and widely known form of cerebrovascular disease is stroke, which claims the lives of nearly 150,000 Americans each year, as well as subarachnoid hemorrhage, vascular dementia, and transient ischemic attack (TIA), also known as 'mini strokes' (NYS, 2022). Although each of these conditions will present as an emergency requiring (in most cases) immediate hospitalization, there are also a range of medicines, as well as behaviors and habits that can be undertaken in order to minimize the risk of such adverse events. These include the use of blood thinners and hypertensive medication, as well as lifestyle factors such as healthy diet, regular exercise, and the avoidance or cessation of smoking and tobacco use.

Unlike stroke, where the culprit exists at the molecular level and cannot be easily recognized even in the abstract, it is far easier for my patients over age 50 to conceptualize the actions that they can take in order to reduce their risk of stroke or other cerebrovascular disease. Particularly notable is the image of clogged arteries; although simplistic and perhaps a little reductive, if you can remind yourself of the deadly threat posed by arteries clogged with fat – especially in terms of increased blood pressure and risk of stroke – you'll be more likely to adhere to a heart-healthy diet (CDC. 2022a). A more in-depth consideration of the types of food and cooking choices which go into a heart-healthy diet are detailed in chapter XX.

(2) *Chronic Respiratory Disease* is another major killer of Americans, with this condition mortally afflicting 150,000 Americans every year. Notable for such diseases as emphysema and COPD, chronic respiratory disease is a blanket term for a wide range of lung diseases, the most common symptoms of which being blockage of airflow and difficulty breathing. Bronchitis and COPD can also result in permanent scarring and other damage to the lungs, but like asthma, the course of emphysema can be reversed through activity and behavioral lifestyle changes (WHO, 2022). Perhaps even more so than the risk of stroke, and certainly more than cancer, it is easy for my patients over 50 to understand this problem and to recognize the potential paths (like quitting smoking, especially) they may take to prevent or slow its progression.

Heart Disease. This work now turns to cardiovascular (heart) disease, which will inform the central focus of the remainder of these recommendations. Heart conditions, when considered in general, include structural problems in the heart, blood clots, and disease which affects the vessels of the heart. Particular types of cardiovascular disease include (1) *coronary artery disease*, which reflects damage or disease in the major vessels of the heart; (2) *high blood pressure*, in which the force of the blood against the walls of the arteries is too high, leading to damage or susceptibility to stroke or heart attack, and (3) *cardiac arrest*, a disastrous condition involving immediate loss of heart function, alongside loss of breathing and consciousness (CDC, 2022a).

Worse than stroke, cardiovascular disease is the leading cause of death in the United States, with this top standing identical among men and women, as well as across all major ethnic groups. Roughly 660,000 Americans die from heart disease each year, or roughly one in four recorded deaths. Distressingly, one person dies of heart disease in the United States every 36 seconds (CDC, 2022a). This topic will be considered in far greater detail in the chapters to come. For now, it is important to indicate that heart disease is the most important health threat which people over 50 must recognize; additionally, unlike cancer but similar to cerebrovascular disease, there are some relatively straightforward health maintenance and preventive health measures which individuals can take to slow the progression of heart disease or to prevent adverse heart events – like heart attack – altogether. Before those measures are considered in detail, it is crucial to also examine additional threat vectors which take advantage not only of ill health, but prey upon poor health-related behaviors and unhealthy behavioral decision making.

Leading Comorbidities. In addition to heart disease and other leading causes of death, there are particular comorbid factors which must be considered. Notably, these are factors, behaviors, and choices which are entirely within the control of the individual, and for which education and motivation represent the only true obstacles. The three leading comorbidities which most influence and exacerbate the threat of the particular causes of death considered above, are tobacco use, poor diet, and physical inactivity.

Previous sections have considered the threat posed by tobacco use and some detail, and this work will consider the *heart healthy diet* in sections to come, so let's touch upon diet and physical activity.

Recent figures from the Bureau of Labor Statistics show that 19.3% (or fewer than one in five) Americans engaged in daily sports or physical exercise (or physical leisure activities) in 2019 (DuCharme, 2018). Although the rate was slightly higher for men than it was for women, both men and women showed abysmally low levels of physical activity. Conversely, such low levels of physical activity translate directly to high levels of sedentary activity, such as sitting in a chair, sitting on the couch or lying down. Such sedentary behavior is directly linked to increased risk of all-cause mortality, including resulting in a doubling of heart disease risk factors and a range of other cardiovascular disease, increasing risk of diabetes, obesity, high blood pressure, osteoporosis, and specific cancers (particularly colon cancer) (CDC, 2022).

Additionally, sedentary lifestyle has been linked to increased rates of anxiety and depression disorders (CDC, 2022). Put simply, exercise and physical activity, no matter the form it takes, are not only associated with a vastly reduced risk of a wide range of disease and disorder, but physical activity can result in a marked improvement to quality of life and mental health.

Preventive Examination, Vaccination, and Healthcare 'Engagement'. The section now turns to one of the most important actions that any individual can take in order to optimize their own health outcomes over age 50. These are preventive health screenings and the prioritization of the individual's overall healthcare 'engagement'. Let's consider health screenings first. Past age 50, it becomes more important than ever to undergo cholesterol, diabetes, and high blood pressure screenings, with the results of each of these applied toward meaningful health and behavioral decisions. Additionally, women older than age 50 should undergo regular osteoporosis and breast cancer screenings, and men over age 40 should undergo colorectal cancer screening.

Vaccinations are also important, including those against pneumococcal viruses, particularly pneumonia, as well as the recently released vaccinations to protect against the novel coronavirus COVID-19 (De Leon et al., 2021). As we age, it becomes more important than ever to remain current with vaccinations and to undergo regular health screenings for a wide range of conditions.

This preventive approach to care management also hinges upon maintaining a certain degree of **engagement with your primary care provider** as well as the other specialist caregivers who you may see to discuss specific problem areas. Although it may be unfortunate to consider, it is not beneficial to ignore health maintenance behaviors, no matter the degree to which you were able to 'get away' with such behaviors in your youth. Now is no time to neglect your health, and in fact, far more benefits, particularly in terms of longevity, can be achieved through taking an active role in your own care. However, as considered in this section, it is important to ensure that the awareness and interest that you have in your own care does not give way to paranoia or hypochondria. Your body is more resilient than it may seem, so it is not useful or conducive to quality of life to worry about every potential health hazard.

When considered in this way, the importance of taking a statistically-driven or 'probabilistic' approach to preventive care past age 50 is revealed to be useful. For instance, a strong example of the probabilistic perspective of preventive care is in the distinction between cancer and heart health screening in old age. In nearly every instance, it is more important for the individual to recognize the threat posed by heart disease than cancer (Cao et al., 2017) This is true for a range of reasons, all of which reflect the wider focus upon prevention in this chapter, and the simple fact that cancer threats are much less 'affected' by behavioral changes than threat of heart disease.

OVERVIEW

This chapter has touched upon a wide range of points which are highly relevant to the health maintenance goals of anyone over age 50. It is never too late to begin a course of preventive care, but this chapter has stressed that it is crucial for the individual to determine the areas of greatest risk to which they are exposed, as well as to recognize certain threats where prevention is not worth the effort. In particular, this chapter has suggested that cancer risks, in particular, do not 'play by the same rules' as other high mortality diagnoses. In particular, heart disease and lung disease are acutely influenced by changes in lifestyle behaviors. By contrast, cancer can afflict individuals whose lifestyles, diets, and behaviors are perfectly conducive to cancer prevention. At the same time, individuals who lead lives of extraordinarily ill health or negative health decisions, may be 'unfairly' spared from a cancer diagnosis. It is for this reason that, despite the high rates of cancer mortality in the United States, it is not reasonable to devote more than a minimal amount of energy toward preventative behavior which focuses upon cancer alone.

Fortunately, many of the same behaviors which have been linked to cancer prevention – though hardly definitively – form the basis for strong recommendations with respect to the prevention of heart disease. Such ideas include the cessation of smoking and particular, as well as an improved diet and a reduction in sedentary behavior or the adoption of exercise and other physical activity. There is no question that the lifestyle changes outlined in this chapter regarding prevention of heart disease are indeed associated with a marked reduction in all-cause mortality. In the United States, where heart disease is astoundingly, tragically common – alongside sedentary lifestyle behaviors – there are a range of behavioral changes which individuals can undertake to achieve a marked reduction in heart disease risk. In doing so, individuals can reduce risk of heart attack, stroke, high blood pressure, and a range of other negative health events associated with increased mortality. In all instances, improved outcomes were also associated with maintaining an active relationship with a primary care provider, getting to doctor's appointments on time, and adhering to medication directives and behavioral recommendations.

Above all these recommendations is the **personal mindset** regarding life and longevity outlined in the chapter to follow. Psychology will be shown to play a strong role in the individual's understanding of their own lifespan, as well as the commitments to good health which they must maintain. In the following chapter we will consider the importance of maintaining a preventive care 'mindset', which can be used to uphold heart healthy behavior over age 50. This work will continue to drive down to its ultimate focus on heart-healthy behavior past age 50, but the chapter to follow will provide a strong psychological basis for maintaining a productive and healthy point of view.

REFERENCES

Cao, B., Bray, F., Beltrán-Sánchez, H., Ginsburg, O., Soneji, S., & Soerjomataram, I. (2017). Benchmarking life expectancy and cancer mortality: global comparison with cardiovascular disease 1981-2010. BMJ, 357.

Centers for Disease Control and Prevention (CDC. 2022). *Cancer data and statistics*. Retrieved from https://www.cdc.gov/cancer/dcpc/data/index.htm

(2022a). *Heart disease facts*. Retrieved from https://www.cdc.gov/heartdisease/facts.htm

(2022b). How to prevent cancer or find it early. Retrieved from https://www.cdc.gov/cancer/dcpc/prevention/index.htm

De-Leon, H., Calderon-Margalit, R., Pederiva, F., Ashkenazy, Y., & Gazit, D. (2021). First indication of the effect of COVID-19 vaccinations on the course of the COVID-19 outbreak in Israel. medRxiv.

DuCharme, J. (2018). Only 23% of Americans Get Enough Exercise, a New Report Says. *Time Magazine*. Retrieved from https://www/time.com/5324940/americans-exercise-physical-activity-guidelines

New York State Department of Health (NYS, 2022). *Heart disease and stroke prevention*. Retrieved from https://www.health.ny.gov/diseases/cardiovascular/heart_disease/

World Health Organization (WHO, 2022). *Chronic respiratory diseases*. Retrieved from https://www.who.int/health-topics/chronic-respiratory-diseases

CHAPTER 4

♥

'THE PREVENTIVE CARE MINDSET' AND HEART HEALTH OVER THE LIFESPAN

HEART HEALTH IS A MATTER of the physical health of the muscle itself, and the need to protect at all costs the efficiency and ability at which the heart performs its one and only task. The heart is the perennial workhorse of the body, pumping blood to your every organ and physical extremity about 100,000 times per day, about 35 million times a year, and over 2.5 billion times in an average lifespan. For most it might be preferable to not consider the sheer amount of work that the heart has to perform in a lifespan. Considered in a certain way, a sense of unease might be unavoidable when bearing in mind the heart's tenuous necessity and vulnerability alongside the rest of the body.

In this chapter, we're really getting down to the 'nitty gritty' of heart health. After all, lifestyle outcomes and optimal habits are only ways of maintaining the longevity of a fist-sized organ called the heart. To expand off the previous chapter, the following chapter will consider ways in which optimal heart-healthy behaviors (such as tobacco use, poor diet, and physical inactivity) are best considered as acute threats to your overall longevity alongside cancer, cardiovascular disease, falls, and osteoporosis. Regular screenings and outcomes-focused behavioral changes also represent critical approaches to optimizing heart health, but some people can often find such behavioral changes difficult to maintain over time, or fall back into old ('non heart-healthy) behaviors over time as a result of losing interest in their doctor's orders. In this chapter, we're going to do a 'deep dive' on the problems of **mindset** which I believe are at the core of every failed diet and which influence every lifestyle of poor heart health.

But while we're getting down to basics, let's get the 'hard part' out of the way too. It might seem obvious, but as people age, the heart ages as well. Over time, heart aging can result in predictable things happening. For instance, over time even as your resting heart rate remains unchanged, increased strain means the heart can't beat as fast when engaging in stressful activity or physical exertion. Arterial stiffness or arteriosclerosis is a common culprit in this common aging-related heart malady, which has been associated with increased rates of high blood pressure, which leads to increased stroke or heart attack risk. That said, government agencies have stressed awareness of common causes of arteriosclerosis for years, and I'd wager that the concept of dietary fatty deposits accumulating on the walls of arteries is well-ingrained in the public imagination. Different types of heart damage over the lifespan can also occur as a result of existing hypertension resulting from cigarette smoking or alcohol use, or from age-related change in the body's electrical system resulting in arrhythmias.

Regardless of your heart-related dietary and other behaviors, overall risk of coronary heart disease, stroke, or heart attack goes up after the age of 65. Ideally – and if there's one bit of practical wisdom you can take from this overview, it's that – as soon as possible (but definitely after the age of 65), **take a behavioral and dietary accounting**, and audit your behaviors and food intake for their heart-healthiness. This plan might seem like an onerous burden which requires an unnecessarily large amount of work. The idea of a full accounting might even conjure up ideas of spreadsheets or ledgers, and I'm here to tell you that yes, a spreadsheet might help. This won't be a simple process, but if viewed in the proper context, undertaking a deeply focused bout of introspection and behavioral accounting might seem a simple, helpful commitment.

What am I talking about? I'll explain, but it's important to 'start from the top'.

Consider the concept of the 'heart lifespan' and of 'heart age.' You might have heard these terms before. You can find simple calculator tools online which use age and overall lifespan an informal and simple shorthand for measuring your heart health risk. An instrument from the Mayo Clinic (2022) allows users to account for such risk, and offers a 'heart age' as a factor of their responses to a survey about lifestyle factors ice diet, smoking, and physical activity. Results which people receive when they plug their lifestyle information into this instrument can be a little startling – its author, the medical doctor Francisco Lopez-Jimenez explains that 'most American' users' 'heart age' is far higher than their 'regular age'. However disturbing, it appears that the heart age calculator provides a useful way to conceptualize the 'longitudinal' health of the heart as a 'lifespan' in its own right. Helpfully, the heart age calculator indicates that overall heart age can be reduced (an indicator of greater heart health) through smoking cessation, regular physical exercise, heart-healthy diet with limited salt, and a host of other metabolism-related recommendations, especially glucose control. We have considered many of these risks already, but it is important to reiterate that heart-healthy behaviors are specific and understandable, as well as attainable with some willpower.

But alongside these common-sensual recommendations, the Mayo Clinic's idea of conceiving of heart health in terms of an overall heart 'lifespan' shines through, for this concept contains a unique wisdom: If the heart is understood to be a 'life' in its own right, it becomes possible to conceive of your responsibility to protect and prolong the life of your own 'heart health,' much the same as you might value strategies to prolong your overall lifespan. Also, I think the reader may agree: The idea of 'heart age' might even be enchanting in a way: On one hand, the concept of a heart age greater than one's own would seem to offer a horrible vision of being 'led' toward death by prematurely-elderly organs. But on the other hand, it offers the idea of improved heart health as a 'fountain of youth', where it is possible to rejuvenate your life and discover a more youthful sense of vigor, through actions as simple as cutting dietary cholesterol.

This is not to disparage the willpower that dieting requires, but the idea of 'heart age' might be especially useful for dieting because it allows you to better-conceptualize the diet as something of great long-term benefit. To help you understand this helpful viewpoint, **the 'eternalist' idea of the self** is useful as a philosophical framing device. Bear with me here: Although the heart grows old over the lifespan, it might be argued that your individual **duty to care** for the heart makes the most sense when you conceive of heart health not only in the context of today, but in terms of total 'lifespan', including the heart's full past and future. Using this idea and – let's say, this meditation aid or thought experiment – might be a little easier said than done, but in my view, the 'lifespan' view of heart health offers a beneficial and 'holistic', whole-life approach to preventive or maintenance care. The associated idea of 'externalism' is uniquely suited to explaining the benefits of this type of thought, and offers an interesting image:

Think of every moment of your life being equally 'real'. This is an image of every moment of your existence, in effect 'happening at the same time.' By taking 'time' out of the equation, eternalist philosophy allows you to see yourself existing as a 'total' lifespan. It remains one where your actions today 'affect' your future health, safety, and peace of mind, but the 'you' who will exist – and the heart beating in the chest of that 'future you' – is *equally* as much you, as you are, and equally as deserving of respect. The same might be said for the 'you' who you used to be (and 'their' heart), because no one would argue that the self you are today (and the circumstances you face today) were *not* influenced by the version of you who you used to be.

This is where reader might need to make a theoretical 'leap': It's useful to conceive off heart healthy behaviors as behaviors that will influence the person you will become tomorrow, because this **is the same idea** which describes the influence you feel as a product of the decisions you made yesterday. By breaking down the walls between today and tomorrow, you can look at **heart health as a lifelong project**.

This is beneficial because if you can see yourself as old and frail, it may trigger the impulse to protect that version of you. If you truly sympathize with yourself in the future, heart-healthy behaviors become (in this 'lifelong' context) a moderate commitment at worst and a pleasure at best.

If I haven't reached you yet, I implore you to **live today with the heart health of yourself in the future in mind**. In fact, if you can master this idea, it can be useful in motivating healthy behavior today. Ultimately, 'eternalism' as a mental framing device for your own lifespan (which also implies the 'heart lifespan') is most useful when used to distance yourself from day-to-day annoyances that accompany diet or heart-healthy behavior changes, and more often in later life. Let's quickly explore the difference between these two ways which a diet or heart-healthy behavior change are motivated.

At age 65, an example person might engage in heart-healthy behaviors because they are informed by their primary care provider that they must do so. So they diet out of a sense of obligation, but the diet doesn't seem to 'take'. Who can't relate to feeling chafed under the onerous terms of a diet? It's no mystery: Even an important heart-related behavioral change like dieting or cholesterol control, if made of a compulsion or under a requirement understood but not felt to be important, is doomed to fail.

But this is where the **airtight diet tip** of the 'eternal' view of the self comes in. In fact, I submit that

NO DIET CAN FAIL

If it is truly motivated by a sense of improving heart health for the *rest of your life*.

I'll admit this idea might seem complicated or perhaps difficult to understand, but I beg the reader to try to step back from your current idea of time for a second. Have you done it? Now, try to envision your life as 'one thing happening once'. Trust me, it's useful. See, to understand this idea might require a re-framing of your sense of self, but I'll bet that your sense of self was already in need of some repair. You're still skeptical?

I'll tell you why:

In the U.S., attitudes around procrastination often celebrate the person putting off whatever job they still have to do, even though it's no secret that 'putting off to tomorrow what you might do today' is irresponsible behavior (nowhere greater than in the province of your health). So why do we do it? To put off an uncomfortable or strenuous task to tomorrow certainly allows for more leisure or pleasure today, but speaking of universal experiences, doesn't procrastination usually turn out for the worse?

After all, who can't relate to the idea of feeling 'abused' by yourself from the day before, whether in the form of a devastating hangover or some burning task which this 'other' you left incomplete? Isn't this an irrational view? But why does it feel so real?

This is where the 'eternal' view of the self is most useful: It helps you to envision behavior and identity not as something which occurs throughout your life, but instead views your every action as contributing to and helping to influence your life (and health, and heart health) *as a whole picture*. Although you can't foresee the future *as such*, this 'whole life' approach to health can help you to better care for your heart health today.

Because it means that your future heart health reflects your actions today.

So what?

Well I'll tell you, the idea of 'heart lifespan' and the 'eternalist' view of the self (where all actions contribute to an overall 'lifespan health') can help people of all ages to effectively sidestep a tricky logical landmine known as **the 'sunk cost' fallacy**.

Now, I'm not about to suggest that it's necessary to view your every decision as pitted against a veritable minefield of logical fallacies and psychological biases or other mental 'blind spots'. To do so would be ruinous to quality of life. But, it may be useful to let at least threat of the sunk cost fallacy inform a 'whole lifespan' view of optimal heart-healthy behaviors. You might have heard of the 'sunk cost' fallacy; sometimes in the face of ever increasingly-bad outcomes, people will continue to 'double down' on the same irrational behavior for the simple but illogical reason that they 'always acted this way.' This behavior appears to have resulted from a primal fear of change resulting in a hard preference for continuing the 'understood' behavior (no matter how sub-optimal) over changing to an optimal approach, especially when the change will be painful.

So rather than facing the problem head-on, psychological victims of the 'sunk cost' fallacy continue to embody certain biases. Worse yet, these biases can make them likelier to move up along the 'escalation of commitment'. This describes situations where already-negative behaviors become catastrophic. Victims of this illogical and sub-optimal fallacy mindset will continue to make the same poor decisions that led to their predicament, and in some cases, with greater 'commitment' of energies and resources. For example, the smoker who spends twenty years gradually building to a pack a day, not only refuses to quit after their first heart attack, but escalates their commitment and smokes two packs a day. These cases are tragic, but even less-urgent poor heart health decisions can be said to represent a 'poor way to run a railroad', in terms of your lifelong health maintenance duty: Eating poorly or smoking because you've always eaten poorly or smoked represents – effectively – **throwing good money after bad**.

No matter the life you lead tomorrow, that person who is you tomorrow is *also you today*, because you will wake up tomorrow to face the consequences of the actions you take today. Though it might be difficult to separate from your 'self' as you exist now, it is also possible to imagine yourself waking up thirty years from now, subject to the consequences of the actions you take today and every day to come. Do you want to wake up in a spry physical form, perhaps fragile like a bird but with a heart of iron, bounding out of bed ready to meet the day? Or will your first thought on waking be regret and discomfort at the ache of an overtaxed and decayed body?

Let's not 'dwell' on the miseries of old age, but I bring up this contrast to highlight the benefit of thinking about catering to the likeliest wishes of your own old age. That is, you must **get in touch with what you will want when you are old**. Ideally such ideas are already informing your actions, but it's important to take a full accounting of your behaviors and physical intake and stress (for instance), so that you can optimize the person you'll become.

Think of such an accounting in terms of paying your proper respects to the very elderly person you might hope to live long enough to become. Or if you prefer, it may be beneficial to important to focus on yourself as a lifelong project made up of behaviors which are not random but focused, constant, and cherished out of sense of timeless obligation. I feel the metaphor of the ceiling of the Sistine Chapel works well here: Its beauty was the product of diligence and a sense of duty so great because it was motivated by a sense of responsibility that existed well outside the comprehension of even its painter. So let me tell you: Personally, I've had enough of modesty, and so should you. You're a masterpiece, and its time you started acting that way. "But how?" you may still ask. You have to see yourself as a permanent work-in-progress, and heart-healthy behaviors not as a painful or difficult obligation, but as the necessary sacrifices to reap the benefits of a kind of 'fountain of youth.' The trick is to start working on heart-healthy behaviors now, with the potential for improvement (and reduced 'heart age') open to all ages, even when an unhealthy heart and painful old age appears 'locked in.'

DISCUSSION

In addition to anticipating the needs of your future self, please do not regret the impropriety or witless abandon of days gone by: The 'whole life' view of heart health works in 'either' direction, meaning that you are also the person you used to be. It is of no use to feel anything toward this past version of you except for sympathy and understanding. If there's nothing you take away from this chapter's diversion into the metaphysical, recognize that that **regret is a useless feeling**. The past cannot be changed. All we have is today and the future to come, and living a life dominated by sadnesses gone by detracts from the very real power of today. There is a Chinese proverb that says: "The best time to plant a tree was 20 years ago. The second best time is now." It's impossible to change decisions that you've already made, but you can treat your decisions today as if some version of you in thirty years is equally alive and valid. Maybe this version of you exists on their deathbed, or maybe they're playing tennis, but I ask you to permit these 'future you' to vote on the actions you take today.

This is where regret can be so painful, because to feel regret is to feel the pain of not having a 'seat at the table' when it comes to your own past decisions. If you can successfully 'transpose' your current understanding of yourself onto the 'self' you will become, you can imagine how they would vote on the decisions you make today.

Giving one's future self a vote in present actions and behaviors represents the 'inverse' of regret: It is the anticipation *and avoidance* of future regret, and the pain that such regret is likely to cause. This is a similar idea as deferring to the voices of your ancestors, but pulls from the vision (albeit imaginary) of wisdom anticipated in your own old age. Ultimately, the importance of this 'change in context' or the 'eternalist' and 'whole life' view of heart and overall lifespan is intended to inform habit formation.

Once heart-healthy behaviors are in place, then there is less of a need to conceptualize the life outside the present orientation. That said, the 'whole-life' view of healthy behaviors is also useful in a multitude of other ways aside from heart health. Once you discover how passionately you may work on behalf of the self you are to become, you may find that such behavior becomes second nature. You are not likely to suffer under this mindset, and following the preventive path of the proverbial diligent ant (rather than the frivolous grasshopper) can certainly lead to much-improved cardiovascular health and the potential for strong 'heart longevity' outcomes as well.

REFERENCES

Carstensen, L. L. (2006). The influence of a sense of time on human development. *Science*, *312*(5782), 1913-1915.

Gofman, J. W., Young, W., & Tandy, R. (1966). Ischemic heart disease, atherosclerosis, and longevity. *Circulation*, *34*(4), 679-697.

Gottlieb, D. J., Yenokyan, G., Newman, A. B., O'Connor, G. T., Punjabi, N. M., Quan, S. F., ... & Shahar, E. (2010). Prospective study of obstructive sleep apnea and incident coronary heart disease and heart failure: the sleep heart health study. *Circulation*, *122*(4), 352-360.

Keech, J. J., Cole, K. L., Hagger, M. S., & Hamilton, K. (2020). The association between stress mindset and physical and psychological wellbeing: Testing a stress beliefs model in police officers. *Psychology & Health*, *35*(11), 1306-1325.

Kubzansky, L. D., & Thurston, R. C. (2007). Emotional vitality and incident coronary heart disease: benefits of healthy psychological functioning. *Archives of general psychiatry*, *64*(12), 1393-1401.

Lopez-Jiminez, F. (2022). Heart age. *The Mayo Clinic*. Retrieved from https://www.mayoclinic.org/diseases-conditions/heart-attack/expert-answers/heart-age/faq-20322777

Quinn, P. K., & Reznikoff, M. (1986). The relationship between death anxiety and the subjective experience of time in the elderly. *The International Journal of Aging and Human Development*, *21*(3), 197-210.

Ronayne, A. (2018). The Influence of a Positive or Negative Mindset on Affect and Heart Rate Variability.

Schweitzer, R. D., Head, K., & Dwyer, J. W. (2007). Psychological factors and treatment adherence behavior in patients with chronic heart failure. *Journal of Cardiovascular Nursing*, *22*(1), 76-83.

Zulfiqar, U., Jurivich, D. A., Gao, W., & Singer, D. H. (2010). Relation of high heart rate variability to healthy longevity. *The American journal of cardiology*, *105*(8), 1181-1185.

♥

CHAPTER 5

MODIFIABLE RISK FACTORS FOR ATHEROSCLEROSIS AND OTHER HEART DISEASE

WE NOW TURN TO THE purpose of this work: Information and advice that can help ensure that your heart (and you!) stay healthy past age 50. Unfortunately, aside from what instruments like stethoscopes and x-ray machines can provide, the question of *what* the heart *is* can loom large in the imagination. I find that knowledge about the heart 'as a thing', and without the social 'baggage' that is attached to the heart as a symbol, can be very useful in instilling heart-healthy behaviors. So what is the heart?

Well, the heart is an organ the size of a clenched fist that sits right between your right and left lungs. As it happens, your left lung is a little bit smaller than your right, in order for your chest cavity to accommodate the heart and the lung in the same space as your right lung occupies. It's blocked by ribs, but if you want to 'touch' your heart, it's three ribs down from your clavicle on the left side, just to the left of the sternum.

BUT WHAT *IS* THE HEART?

This is where metaphor comes in handy. First, the heart is like an electric pump and generator; with each beat, the heart outputs 1.33 watts of energy, equivalent to the electricity it takes to run a lightbulb. This might not sound like a lot, but multiply that energy output and physical force by the **3.3 billion** times that the heart beats in an average lifetime. This way, we can recognize the heart as a marvel of stamina and physical endurance. It is a pump that can never cease! Unsurprisingly, the passage of time (and the forces of gravity, essentially) result in a lifetime of 'wear and tear' on this internal 'blood pump.' This reasoning reminds us that as much as it may seem like it must, the heart cannot pump forever. Indeed, like all vital organs, the health of the heart is absolutely indispensable both to life (*and quality of life*) past age 50, meaning it's absolutely fundamental that you pay attention to its proper running. In fact, I suggest you frame an old Valentine's Day card and display it on your desk or in the living room.

Your visitors will think your conspicuous bright red cartoon heart is cute or romantic, but *you'll* know what it really means.

I'm serious!

Alongside the thought experiment in Chapter 4, I am a firm believer that 'idle' heart-unhealthy behaviors resulting from carelessness can be reduced by re-framing and metaphor.

Try acting like the heart is a cherished member of the family – framed picture and all! This exercise helps us on a daily basis to **remember that the heart is there at all**. Because it is a part of our bodies that we'll be lucky to never see with our eyes or feel with our hands, it's easy to forget that it's there. But we must! Even if to confront this fact is to recognize (all too importantly) that we are all mortal, we must remember that our 'allotted' 3.3 billion heartbeats is not an entitlement but an average. It's hard to hear, but for someone to refuse to quit smoking or to avoid sedentary behavior, or – as is also discussed below – to continue behaviors which worsen arteriosclerotic or hypertensive symptoms, is for them to *abuse* their heart. In this instance, personification of the heart helps to emphasize its vulnerability and dependence on your preventive care, and also its admirable 'human' qualities of lifelong service and single-minded devotion to the (and I'm sure you'll agree) highly important assignment of *keeping you alive.*

If you think of the heart not as a 'part of you' but as a small animal (say, a rodent on a treadmill), the reflexive affection you'd feel for that creature just might extend to behaviors to make its life of unending toil a little bit less taxing.

Here's another one: The difference between a healthy heart and an unhealthy one is like the difference between a clean and a dirty machine (which must _never_ stop). Fatty acid deposits throughout the heart and circulatory system due to atherosclerosis, and general muscle deterioration due to any combination of age, inactivity, or gravity will result in a thinner and weaker heart that pumps less blood through the body with each cardiac cycle. The heart of the unhealthy person is 'working' just as hard (in the sense that this cycle produces 1.33 watts of energy with each beat), but it must pump more times in a minute in order to fully oxygenate the cells of the body.

A heart which only needs to pump 45 times in a minute can be thought of as a clean, efficient machine, like a new car. (Don't worry; only people in the very best of cardiovascular health have resting heart rates that low.)

But with the 'heart as car' idea, tachycardia (or high resting heart rate) can be analogized to the running of an inefficient, old car. Higher risk for hypertension or heart attack or stroke can be thought of as more common in hearts like 'rust bucket' cars that haven't been serviced in decades. Like these cars buck and pop and seize and send up clouds of black smoke, but continues to drive, the unhealthy heart also continues to run, but unlike the car, it offers few advance warnings of decline. Unfortunately, the body only 'alerts' the conscious mind to poor heart health if an adverse heart event *is occurring*. It's unfortunate, but the body hasn't evolved means of alerting us to progressive organ deterioration or weakening, so we must assume that our hearts are the same as anyone else's, and assume a proactive preventive health perspective.

One last metaphor, before we get into the 'nuts and bolts' of heart-unhealthy behaviors to avoid. We all know that bad habits affect more than just our own health, but affect the health, peace of mind, and ultimately, the longevity, of our loved ones and of entire families. Try thinking of the heart as a treasured family member *alongside* your other cherished relatives. Neglecting the heart is to expose the family to financial and emotional burdens which *will* result, given enough time. Your heart is the 'seat' of your wellbeing, much like the mind, but it asks comparatively little of you in return. So, what we earn from paying the least degree of attention to our heart habits, is a healthy heart which allows our family members to worry a little less. "After all," your loved ones might say of you someday soon, "[his or her] heart is healthy as can be." I find that deep down, we want our loved ones to be free from worry. But to neglect the heart is to cause your family to worry about your welfare the same as if you were unable or unwilling to care for a sibling or child. It's important stuff, and it deserves this level of gravity.

HEART DISEASE AND HEART-UNHEALTHY BEHAVIORS TO AVOID

Before we get into the heart-healthy behaviors to adopt, it's important to go down the list of common risk factors for atherosclerosis – the deposition of fatty acid plaque on the inside of the arteries – which is the most common risk factor for heart disease or adverse cardiac event. Atherosclerosis is highly common, with 3 million cases diagnosed in the U.S. each year, and it can be a chronic condition even when 'stent' surgeries and other invasive methods are used to clear the plaque from arterial walls. Atherosclerosis is a 'hardening' of the arteries, caused by fatty deposits, and in some cases it can become so acute that the arteries can be blocked by blood clots. One of the most efficient ways of causing such a 'hardening' of the arteries is through **cigarette smoking**. Although I am overjoyed at the dropping rates of cigarette smoking I've witnessed in the U.S. in my lifetime, I wish that these foul and poisonous 'luxury' goods were banned altogether. Perhaps more can find the energy to quit if the mechanism of cigarette-caused heart disease was better-known, so let's review the effect that cigarettes have on the heart:

First, inhalation of nicotine and carbon monoxide damages the endothelium, the membrane that lines the inside of the heart and blood vessels. Endothelial cells regulate vascular relaxation and contraction by releasing hormones and enzymes which set off and correct for blood clotting, arterial immune function and the adhesion properties of thrombocytes (or 'clotting platelets'). Damaging these complex systems on the inside of the arteries can result in severe negative effects on the sympathetic nervous system. While there is little question that the effects of nicotine on the sympathetic system are "transient and stimulant" at first, cigarette smoking can result in a "depressant" effect over time as nicotine's arterial damage (as well as damage to other "organs involved with nicotine action") increases (Leone et al., 2012).

Eventually, after many years of cigarette smoking, damage to nervous tissue and impaired arterial immune function can result in a greater risk for developing plaque buildup on the walls of the arteries. This is because the arteries are no longer as efficient at 'protecting' themselves from such buildup through enzymatic and immune action. Carbon monoxide, the other key toxin to which cigarette smokers are exposed, is a "colorless, odorless and tasteless gas with high and potentially lethal toxicity", which links with hemoglobin (with which it has "chemical affinity"), in the blood (Leone et al., 2012). This results in oxygen being replaced in hemoglobin by carbon monoxide. This chemical reaction leads to the creation of carboxyhemoglobin, leading to both the carbon monoxide and the carboxyhemoglobin poisoning threatening tissue hypoxia and cellular metabolism impairment. Carbon monoxide poisoning can kill in short order (like in an unventilated space with a gas leak), but when inhaled in small amounts over many years, it can result in the same sort of progressive damage to the arteries as nicotine, by periodic, acute 'minor' hypoxia. But in any case:

Quit Smoking

If you skimmed the paragraphs above, let **quit smoking** be the lesson you take away from this chapter. Get help if you need it, or try nicotine replacement therapy (NRT), but as much as for the health of your heart as your lungs, I implore you to quit smoking. The recommendation barely in 'second place' is to reduce sedentary behaviors. In fact, stand up. I'm serious! Stand up right now, and stretch your arms to the ceiling. Touch your toes. Do one 'jumping jack'. *Anything.* Your heart will thank you.

Cardiac risks from sedentary behavior are at a bit of a 'crossroads' at the moment: On one hand, people's awareness of the threat posed by sedentary behavior has never been higher, but the *mechanism* of this risk – I fear – remains poorly-understood, leading to enthusiasm to change behaviors becoming difficult to sustain. Let's review: Sedentary lifestyle is characterized by a lack of movement, which results in a reduced demand on the heart and organs. It may seem odd, but the human body did not evolve to sit in chairs or on couches for extended periods of time. Your body was meant to be upright *and to move* for many hours each day, and if you sat, it was on the ground and some exertion was necessary in order to stand up again.

As a brief aside, an enduring anthropological theory suggests that our bodies evolved to engage in 'persistence hunting', whereby early humans would spend many hours tracking big game animals across the African savanna until the animals collapsed from overheating and exhaustion. Our highly advanced 'radiator' (sweating) is often taken as evidence of this 'specialization.' In any case, whether or not distance running represents our 'biological destiny', I think you'll agree that the body doesn't seem to 'enjoy' sedentary behavior as much as the mind. Minor aches and pains can result when you sit for a long period of time, or worse, tissue injury can result, and in extreme cases – like in those unfortunate people on long flights who forget to get up and stretch every few hours – a fatal embolism can result.

Perhaps unsurprisingly, these threats align closely with the heart risk behaviors which sedentary lifestyle poses. So what are the **heart risks of sedentary behavior**, specifically? They are a multi-pronged threat: Reduced physical demand on the heart can result in blood moving more slowly throughout the body. This will often result in a greater likelihood of fatty acid buildup on arteries. Additionally, sedentary lifestyle results in a decreased capacity to process fats; "your body's production of lipoprotein lipase", an arterial enzyme important to fat processing, "drops by about 90 percent" when you sit (Beaumont, 2022). Sitting can also cause "insulin resistance", a risk factor for obesity and type-2 diabetes, both of which increase heart disease risk (Beaumont, 2022). Worse yet, the skeleton weakens after extended periods of sedentary activity, and the muscles can atrophy, *including the heart*. Muscle weakness and atrophy can result in a heart which is not as muscular as a healthy heart, leading to reduced cardiovascular efficiency which exacerbates the other cardiovascular risk factors considered.

Lastly, **reduce lifestyle stress**. The heart is a muscle which evolved during our evolutionary past as wild animals, and the fossil record shows that it hasn't changed substantially at least 100,000 years. Even in modern society with its social graces and laws against violent crime, stress can result in a 'fight or flight' response. Though it seems like a 'vestige', adrenaline and cortisol flooding the bloodstream at a moment of acute stress can result in a safe resolution to an unsafe situation. Certainly there are none among us who would wish to not become extremely alert and aroused in an emergency – such as when escaping (or helping others to escape) from a burning building – but stress reactions can also be 'counterproductive' in some instances.

Navigating the complexity of the office or other social environment, or dealing with rude people, can cause stress because the body – on a 'deep down' level – often cannot tell the difference between a trivial confrontation and one which threatens our survival and reproduction potential. Hence stress and 'fight or flight' remains central to our evolutionary, instinctual 'bag of tricks.' Unfortunately, the body and heart were not prepared for the realities of modern human life, often with its perpetual 'low-level' stress (like that which people feel as a result of a difficult economic circumstance, or when a loved one is in the hospital). In these situations, far more so than in the cardiovascular system of an ancestor who had to outrun a water buffalo, stress effects can be cumulative over time. For instance, lifestyle stress at a low or 'constant' level can result in tissue inflammation, which results in high blood pressure and lower 'good' cholesterol (HDL). Additionally, excess worry can result in poor sleep. Poor sleep means people are less likely to exercise and more likely to make heart-unhealthy eating or lifestyle behaviors. Stress compounds sedentary behavior risk, and the image of the stressed smoker continues to endure. Future chapters will consider means by which this goal can be achieved, but reducing lifestyle stress remains one of the most useful choices that you can make to reduce heart disease risk exposure.

Each of the above recommendations aligns with the reduction in a range of specific heart-unhealthy conditions, often comorbid with stroke, heart attack, or cardiac ischemia (a blockage which results in reduced supply of oxygen, often unnoticed by the victim). These 'intermediate' risk factors include **high blood cholesterol** (also known as hypercholesterolemia) which limits blood flow and can increase stroke or heart attack risk, as is **high blood concentration of triglycerides** (hypertriglyceridemia), a condition traditionally associated with liver and pancreas problems, but which is now known to adversely affect the heart and lead to higher likelihood of occurring alongside diabetes and obesity. Notably, **hypertension** is a major precursor of stroke and heart attack, with high blood pressure resulting from stress or heart damage over time, placing greater strain on the heart's ability to pump blood and exposing the individual to greater heart disease risk. Heart disease can also result from **lipid imbalance** (dyslipidemia), which causes a host of complex risk factors which exacerbate risk of atherosclerosis. **Obesity** is another major risk factor, manifesting in the form of heart 'enlargement' (a combination of atrial and ventricular enlargement) which results in atherosclerosis, and **diabetes mellitus (especially type 2)**, which can damage the blood vessels as well as the nerves that control the heart and blood vessels. Over time, this sort of tissue damage can lead to heart disease, and the development of heart disease at a younger age than people who do not have diabetes.

However, each of these 'secondary' risk factors can be reduced through heart-healthy prevention behaviors which stress the importance of **quitting smoking, reducing sedentary behavior, and reducing lifestyle stress.** Only the first of these is a 'definitive' recommendation (to quit smoking), with the other two matters consisting of actions in matters of 'degrees.' You need not purchase a standing desk, for instance, when it's likely more cost-effective and just as healthy when working from home or watching TV, to set a timer to stand and stretch every 45 minutes. Similarly, there are other simple 'fixes' to reduce stress, such as meditation and other self-soothing and calming behaviors.

The heart, I have found, is extremely accepting and easy to please. So long as it is not being stifled with carbon monoxide and clogged with plaque (or forced to beat faster than it needs to for longer periods of time than the stressful events to which it evolved to react), it stays happy. Using the metaphor of family member or beloved pet might also help to 'contextualize' your heart-healthy behaviors as well. Don't be afraid to have fun with it; the goal is to build a relationship with your heart to motivate heart-healthy behavior from an emotional point of view. Although it's possible to motivate healthy change behaviors from a 'logical' perspective (and remind oneself of facts that can be gleaned from posters in doctor's offices), this strategy neglects the power of the imagination. Do not hesitate to 'enlist' your emotional, imaginative side when it comes to motivating heart-healthy behavior. The next chapter will explore lifestyle and other decisions you can make to fully 'improve' your heart health. That said, none of the 'positive' changes work without the 'negative' actions outlined in this chapter, so please pay strong attention to the three lifestyle change recommendations discussed here.

REFERENCES

American Heart Association (2022). Chronic stress can cause heart trouble. Retrieved from https://www.heart.org/en/news/2020/02/04/chronic-stress-can-cause-heart-trouble

Beaumont Heart Clinic (2022). *How Sitting Too Much Can Lead to Heart Disease.*

Retrieved from https://www.beaumont.org/health-wellness/blogs/how-sitting-to-much-can-lead-to-heart-disease

Better Health (2021). Heart explained. Retrieved from https://www.betterhealth.vic.gov.au/health/conditionsandtreatments/heart

Centers for Disease Control and Prevention (CDC, 2022). *How Does Sleep Affect Your Heart Health?* Retrieved from https://www.cdc.gov/bloodpressure/sleep.htm

Key Step (2022). Discover the Importance of Self-Empathy. Retrieved from https://www.keystepmedia.com/importance-self-empathy/

Kirn, T. (2019). Opinion: The Persistent Myth of Persistence Hunting. Retrieved from https://undark.org/2019/10/03/persistent-myth-persistence-hunting/

Leone A. How and why chemicals from tobacco smoke can induce a rise in blood pressure. World J Pharmacol 2012; 1(1): 10-20 [DOI: 10.5497/wjp.v1.i1.10]

National Heart, Lung, and Blood Institute (2019). How Smoking Affects the Heart and Blood Vessels. Retrieved from https://www.nhlbi.nih.gov/health/heart/smoking

CHAPTER 6

OPTIMIZING HEART HEALTH PAST AGE 50

Let's start with the most important stuff: **If you've had a heart attack**, you can expect to be prescribed medications that you will have to take for the rest of your life. Casting aside the causes of the heart attack in the first place, *having* a heart attack means heart damage and even 'simply' surviving a heart attack means long-term damage to the arteries and heart muscle, or an arrhythmia which impairs the heart to pump blood, and increases risk of stroke and kidney disorders. Surviving a heart attack can also increase risk of peripheral arterial disease (PAD), which also results from the buildup of fatty plaque in the arteries (atherosclerosis) directly prior to myocardial infarction. The conditions which lead to a heart attack can result in increased risk of further damage to the heart and other organs, and cause an increased risk of death.

(Sorry! Trust me, we're going somewhere with this happy reminder. For the most part, **this chapter is about heart medication**.)

Readers who have had a heart attack are likely to have been prescribed a whole host of heart medicines, including anticoagulants, statins, beta-blockers and ACE inhibitors, but even a combination of medication and 'lifestyle' factors – such as exercise and healthful eating with a strong focus on reducing cholesterol, and trying to limit stress – may not be enough to prevent **loss of quality of life** after a heart attack.

As much as the mind and soul can feel limitless, the negative physical patterns of life can 'accumulate', with arterial plaque only one (highly vivid) example of the 'toll' which time and age can take on the body. But back to my heart attack survivors: you need to keep consistent with your medications, and try your best to remain compliant with all recommendations and advice from your cardiologist or primary care provider, and if you feel you can't do this, you must see to it that your concerns are addressed.

Your life may depend on it!

But let's say that you haven't had a heart attack, and don't 'plan on it' either. Medications to prevent heart attack and prolonging the heart's lifespan can also be part of a heart-healthy lifestyle plan after age 50.

Common medicines prescribed for this purpose include:

(1) **Anticoagulants**. These are often known as 'blood thinners', but they don't actually make the blood 'thinner'; instead, anticoagulants chemically interrupt the process involved in the formation of blood clots, leading to the prevention of blood clotting or the prevention of existing clots from getting larger. Warfarin, rivaroxaban (Xarelto), and apixaban (Eliquis) are the most common of these, and can be taken as tablets without continual blood testing. Why are blood thinners necessary? It may be helpful to think of a blood clot as similar to the plaque that causes myocardial infarction: In both cases there is a blockage in the arterial walls, but where plaque is caused by dietary factors, blood clots are triggered by the immune system. No one would ever argue that blood clotting isn't beneficial in general, but when it happens within the arteries, **clots can be deadly.** When normally-beneficial immune blood platelets stick to the walls of the arteries, they can form a 'plug' that impairs blood flow. If untreated, the clot can grow over time, resulting not only in the accumulation of platelets, but clots in strands of a material called fibrin that form a 'net' upon which platelets accumulate.

Direct oral anticoagulants (DOACs) stop clots growing, but can impair the body's ability make fibrin, the protein which forms the 'mesh' or 'net' of the clot. This medicine carries significant and uncomfortable side effects, most of which involve bleeding: Nosebleeds, prolonged bleeding from a cut, bleeding gums, or worse, can result from anticoagulants. Use of anticoagulants can also cause uncertainty in blood testing, and can interfere with assessment of drug levels and the determination of safe drug levels for major surgery. In other cases, anticoagulants can result in kidney failure (and 'renal dependence' or requiring dialysis). Put simply, anticoagulants are beneficial because they block the immune response, but they are also detrimental for the same reason.

What else can you take? How about (2) **Statins**? These medications lower the levels of low-density lipoproteins (LDL, or 'bad' cholesterol) in the blood, the buildup of which causes arterial plaque buildup and atherosclerosis. Medicines such as lovastatin (Mevacor) or pitavastatin (Livalo) work by reducing the amount of cholesterol the liver makes, and by helping the liver remove LDL (that is, excess or 'waste') cholesterol from the blood. **Statins result in a reduced risk for stroke and heart disease. Full stop.**

Anyway, to determine whether you'd benefit from statins, we need to know your LDL cholesterol levels. These can be determined by blood test. Actually, yearly cholesterol testing is recommended past age 50, but I assume you knew that already, and that I don't have to tell you that a good level of LDL cholesterol is anything less than **100 milligrams per deciliter (mg/dl)**, and that if your level of LDL cholesterol is that low, then you probably don't have to take statins, except for prevention. However, if blood testing shows that your levels of LDL cholesterol is higher than 150 (or as high as 200) mg/dl, then statins are probably indicated as a therapeutic intervention.

Boy! It sure seems that statins are the bee's knees! Seeing that statins prevent heart attack and stroke, **shouldn't everyone take statin medicines?**

The answer is complicated. You see, statins prevent further adverse events once they have occurred (after you've had the heart attack). But if not directly indicated by cholesterol levels, then statins are not necessarily beneficial from what I like to call a 'quality of life' perspective, especially if you're just trying to prevent your 'first' heart attack. This is why it is so important to focus on lifestyle and intake to prevent high LDL cholesterol buildup from impairing heart function in the first place.

Hey – hey. Don't get me wrong. I love statins.

Statins are astonishing medicines which have saved thousands of lives! Maybe tens of thousands!

But the side effects caused by statins are often so uncomfortable and disruptive that people prescribed statins can become reluctant to take them. No question, the side effects are bad: Digestive problems and mental 'fuzziness', and prolonged muscle pain which can come on as a soreness, or as a tiredness or weakness in the muscles. Such muscle pain has been reported by a wide range of individuals prescribed statins, and to interfere with activities of daily living (although somewhat negated through 'nocebo' testing (Moon et al., 2021)). In some rare cases, statins have been linked to major muscle damage called rhabdomyolysis, which can cause severe muscle pain, kidney failure or even death. Statins have also been linked to liver damage, though such damage can be prevented by liver enzyme testing for compatibility prior to prescription.

Statins have also been linked to increased blood glucose levels and with increased risk of developing type-2 diabetes.

Last but surely not least, neurological side effects have been reported with statins, including the 'fuzziness' from above (also known as 'brain fog', it presents as memory difficulties, poor mental clarity, and the inability to focus). The FDA labels all statins with warnings that some people have developed memory loss or confusion while taking statins for common heart-healthy prevention.

Horror story, right? Hold on, it get worse.

Don't forget to t**ake your statins if they're prescribed**, but don't ignore the potential disruption these meds can cause your quality of life, and how such disruption affects your behavior. <u>Now, you might be able to get off the bus right here:</u> If you've been careful with your heart, then your levels of LDL cholesterol may not be high enough to justify the use of statins, so you don't have to worry about their side effects.

And even if you have high cholesterol, then it is not essential to take statins. Talk to your doctor openly about your concerns about statin side effects; it is likely that you can reach some appropriate care plan that takes your concerns into account.

With all that said – **if you've been prescribed statins and the side effects are too much to handle, <u>don't stop taking them without talking to your doctor.</u>**

I've seen it too many times: A patient will survive a heart attack or stroke, some condition for which statins are highly recommended, and then I won't hear from them for some time. After a while, they may report difficulty taking their statins, or even that they are overwhelmed by side effects; in some cases, the patient and I were are able to find additional medicines that helped minimize what is usually muscle pain, but not always.

Sadly (and more than once a heart disease patient might 'fall off the radar', only to resurface after they'd had another heart attack. Although the causes were varied in every case, the 'common denominator' was often that these patients had stopped taking their statins as a result of acute side effects, and hadn't told anyone.

So please, I implore you: Don't 'just stop' taking your meds.

<u>Believe me, I get it:</u> To stop taking a medicine that causes pain *today* on the off chance that you *won't* have a heart attack or stroke at some point in the future, feels like the height of madness. Also, I understand: to stop taking meds which cause side effects can be a relief, and such a relief can be intoxicating. But in the unlikely chance that this paragraph describes your behavior, then please, please, you must talk to your doctor.

Anyway, what other medicines can you take to keep your heart healthy?

How about (3) **Beta blockers** and **ACE Inhibitors?** I'm sure you've heard of these, but what are they? First, beta blockers like metoprolol (Lopressor) are also known as beta-adrenergic blocking agents, These are medicines which block the effects of the hormone epinephrine – and no doubt you've heard of epinephrine, at least by its 'fun' name, **adrenaline**. By blocking the function of the 'fight or flight' response the heart is allowed to beat more slowly and with less force. This reduces blood pressure, and can benefit those with irregular heartbeat or high blood pressure, especially after a heart attack. They also reduce anxiety, tremors, and migraine, and are offered rather diuretics ('water pills') in some cases. Beta blockers also because weight gain and cold hands and feet, and may result in shortness of breath, or depression. Beta blockers reduce the 'potency' of the body's adrenaline/'fight or flight' response, so have also been linked to neurological side effects like drowsiness, lethargy, and other sleep disorders. In certain acute cases, beta blockers have been implicated in nightmares and hallucinations. These sort of neurological side effects like confusion or means that side effects must be monitored and preventive use of medicines as prescribed must be ensured over time.

ACE inhibitors prevent an enzyme in the body from producing angiotensin II, a hormone that narrows blood vessels (and is functionally 'used' by the body to raise blood pressure in the veins and vessels of the heart). They offer similar benefits as beta blockers, but focus on the muscles of the heart and not the adrenaline pathway. In both cases, ACE inhibitors relax and 'open' the heart, resulting in reduced physical pressure on the bloodstream and flow.

Like beta blockers, ACE inhibitors like benazepril (Lotensin) carry a range of side effects that can be unpleasant to endure. Side effects of ACE inhibitors include a dry, irritating cough, dizziness or light-headedness, elevated blood potassium (which can result in the kidney disorder hyperkalemia), angioedema (swelling), and even renal dependence (kidney failure) through inhibited kidney vasoconstriction. Because these side effects are either minor or are determined only by blood test, patients are less likely to stop taking ACE inhibitors against medical advice than to discontinue beta blockers or statins, but any discontinuance behavior against medical advice is still discouraged.

LIFESTYLE DECISIONS AND BEHAVIORS

I hope that the reader has recognized that the 'take away' from the previous section is that the most common medicines to treat heart disease or prevent heart attack or stroke can be a 'mixed bag.' Each of the types of medicines evaluated above has a host of systemic and acute side effects. These can either harm the body quietly, or cause pain and irritation to the person attempting to ward off heart disease. For individuals who take these medicines, ensuring long-term compliance can be difficult.

Is there another way?

Sort of. See, each of us might benefit from heart medicines on a preventive regimen, depending on the degree to which we are at risk. However, after a certain age, the idea of 'relative risk' becomes somewhat 'academic'. After age 50, it's most realistic to simply plan for the breakdown of the heart, or at least fully recognize the necessity of caring for the heart through one's everyday actions. Now those actions can **and often must** include adhering to a regime of prescribed medication including some of the meds considered above. But in most cases, you must remember that medicine is not a 'magic bullet', and heart health is not a matter of simply 'remembering to take your pills.'

Instead, there are two key ways to optimize heart health.

Sadly, if you've read this far expecting to learn some secret and heretofore unknown behavioral key to heart health, you may be disappointed:

See, besides meds, heart health requires **exercise and healthy eating.**

Let's review. (1) **Recommended levels of exercise** (150 minutes of moderate-intensity physical activity and 2 days of some sort of muscle strengthening activity) leads to a wide range of heart health benefits. These include increasing high-density lipoprotein (HDL) (or 'good' cholesterol) and better filtering of unhealthy triglycerides from the blood, leading to more efficient blood flow and reducing risk for cardiovascular disease. It's just that simple. Additional benefits from exercise include reduced risk of stroke, high blood pressure, anxiety, depression, and even arthritis; over time, exercise leads to reduced body weight and your *new, thinner body* causes less strain your bones and the organs, especially the heart. Exercise also improves cognitive function, and has even been associated with an *all-cause reduction in the risk of death.* This means that:

IF YOU EXERCISE REGULARLY, YOU REDUCE YOUR CHANCES OF DYING FROM LITERALLY EVERYTHING.

Your body craves exercise, and to deny the body exercise is to increase your health risk exposure, not least when it comes to the risk of heart disease. Also, if you exercise, it is less likely that you'll have to take any of the medicines considered in the section above, nor put yourself through the pain of the side effects which they cause.

(2) **What about healthful eating?** The American Heart Association recommends a dietary pattern that includes a wide assortment of fruits and vegetables, whole grains, low-fat dairy (like skim milk and low-fat cheese), poultry and fish (without the skin), as well as using nuts, legumes, and non-tropical vegetable oils for cooking.

Also try oats and barley, dark leafy greens, beets, and other vegetables.

Unfortunately, if you haven't been much of a 'vegetable person' in your life, age 50 is the perfect time to start. Think of it as a challenge, not simply to 'endure' a diet higher in legumes, vegetables, and lean meat, but to discover ways to make such a diet palatable or even enjoyable.

You may note that these recommendations do not include red meat or fatty proteins, but this isn't too much of a 'hard and fast' rule: Think of it this way. If heart healthy foods weren't a 'staple' of your diet before, <u>it's time to feed yourself foods that make your heart happy</u>. This isn't to say you may never eat red meat again (unless you've survived a heart attack, then you may consider it). This is to say that following a heart-healthy preventive diet means you should probably save the fatty steak for a special occasion. The point is to ensure your heart is not being *threatened* by your diet. You must strive to ensure most of the food you eat is heart-healthy, but only you know what you can tolerate or how important rich, fatty food is to your quality of life.

This means that if you need to have a 'cheat day' to eat healthfully six days each week, so be it, just stick to a heart-healthy diet plan for the long-haul. Make no mistake, however: **Green leafy vegetables like spinach, kale, collards, as well as almonds and walnuts, and fish like salmon, mackerel, tuna, and sardines, and fruits like strawberries, blueberries, cherries, and oranges, <u>prevent inflammation</u>**, and reduced inflammation prevents risk of cardiovascular disease. It's a simple connection, and verified. You would be very wise to ensure that these foods become a staple of your diet, even if you have to bribe yourself with a morsel of steak on Sundays.

Last but not least: (3) **Heart health depends on limiting stress**, and in **optimizing mental, social, and emotional health**. This is not as difficult as it sounds. Reducing stress can be improved by exercise such as yoga, but also personal and spiritual practices such as the giving of thanks, the act of meditation or prayer, deep breathing, pleasurable activities like listening to music or being in nature, interacting with a pet or loved one, and by protecting personal and professional boundaries.

Optimizing social, and emotional health can result from thinking before acting, trying to connect with others, expressing your feelings in a healthy way, and by trying to remain positive. Most important of all, heart health benefits from finding purpose in life, because self-motivated action and purpose can lead to behavioral benefits in the form of greater discipline or adherence to physician recommendations. Overall, the three recommendations in this section (healthful eating, exercise, and reducing stress) are not necessarily going to prevent your having to take some of the medications considered in the first section. However, neglecting the three factors in this section will mean a much-increased likelihood of having to take heart medicine, and of having to endure their complex or painful side effects. **Why not change your behaviors today**, to avoid the pain and discomfort of having to endure heart medicine side effects in the future?

Cheers! ☺

REFERENCES

Bicket, D. P. (2002). Using ACE inhibitors appropriately. American family physician, 66(3), 461.

Boehm, J. K., Chen, Y., Koga, H., Mathur, M. B., Vie, L. L., & Kubzansky, L. D. (2018). Is optimism associated with healthier cardiovascular-related behavior? Meta-analyses of 3 health behaviors. Circulation research, 122(8), 1119-1134.

Gonsalves, W. I., Pruthi, R. K., & Patnaik, M. M. (2013, May). The new oral anticoagulants in clinical practice. In Mayo Clinic Proceedings (Vol. 88, No. 5, pp. 495-511). Elsevier.

Harter, K., Levine, M., & Henderson, S. O. (2015). Anticoagulation drug therapy: a review. Western Journal of Emergency Medicine, 16(1), 11.

Jafar, T. H., Stark, P. C., Schmid, C. H., Landa, M., Maschio, G., De Jong, P. E. (2003). Progression of chronic kidney disease: the role of blood pressure control, proteinuria, and angiotensin-converting enzyme inhibition: a patient-level meta-analysis. Annals of internal medicine, 139(4), 244-252.

Maron, D. J., Fazio, S., & Linton, M. F. (2000). Current perspectives on statins. Circulation, 101(2), 207-213.

Moon, J., Cohen Sedgh, R., & Jackevicius, C. A. (2021). Examining the nocebo effect of statins through statin adverse events reported in the food and drug administration adverse event reporting system. Circulation: Cardiovascular Quality and Outcomes, 14(1), e007480.

Moosmann, B., & Behl, C. (2004). Selenoprotein synthesis and side-effects of statins. The Lancet, 363(9412), 892-894.

Schroder, K. E., & Schwarzer, R. (2005). Habitual self-control and the management of health behavior among heart patients. Social science & medicine, 60(4), 859-875.

Sirtori, C. R. (2014). The pharmacology of statins. Pharmacological research, 88, 3-11.

Sinzinger, H., Wolfram, R., & Peskar, B. A. (2002). Muscular side effects of statins. Journal of cardiovascular pharmacology, 40(2), 163-171.

Stancu, C., & Sima, A. (2001). Statins: mechanism of action and effects. Journal of cellular and molecular medicine, 5(4), 378-387.

Wiysonge, C. S., Bradley, H. A., Volmink, J., Mayosi, B. M., & Opie, L. H. (2017). Beta-blockers for hypertension. Cochrane database of systematic reviews, (1).

CHAPTER 7

♥

MENTAL HEALTH AND STRESS AND HEART HEALTH IN OLD AGE

Now that we've considered the physical aspects of heart health as they can manifest in impediments to heart health past age 50, it is important to consider mental health as well. I am of the belief that mental health is the most important aspect of overall health, but it is often 'overlooked' by individuals who fail to recognize the connection between mental health (that is, the sense of 'wellbeing' constituting the absence of disorder) and heart health. What's the connection? I think you might agree, that the connection between mental and heart health is in stress, with stress resulting in damage (or the potential for damage) to the heart that mere exercise and pharmaceutical interventions cannot circumvent. So let's talk about stress, and therapeutic techniques found to reduce stress, especially past age 50.

The following chapter provides a comprehensive overview of the links between stress and heart health. To this end, it is necessary to 'break down' what modern science is saying about stress; in some cases, 'common wisdom' may be sufficient, but this book is about improving life and health past age 50, so we'll start by finding the scientific consensus on incidence or perceived stress as this factor influences or otherwise causes greater risk of ill heart health. Once this is established, this chapter will consider what modern science is saying about reducing stress and reducing the acute threat that it poses to the health of the heart and overall health, past age 50.

SO WHAT IS STRESS?

Stress (or worry, or strain) is a reaction to feeling threatened or otherwise being put under pressure. Whether such pressure is physical, environmental, workplace, or social in nature, reactions to such pressures differ from person to person, but in general, acute stress is only useful when it comes to helping you overcome an immediate and pressing obstacle (such as being chased by a wild animal). Such stress is not necessarily detrimental to your heart health. However, the stressors (events or factors that cause stress) of the modern world aren't always or even usually things that threaten our survival. When was the last time you were chased by a tiger?

No, in the modern world, our stressors tend to be more abstract and emotional than that. We worry about things like grocery bills and mortgage payments, or worry over our own livelihoods or those of our loved ones. Day-to-day stressors aren't usually life-threatening either; they often involve little more than unpleasant interactions with other people, or having to endure situations in which one feels as if they are being imposed upon, especially in the workplace. These modern stressors are somewhat abstract as well, meaning that they are partially the result of the imagination. In some instances, stress can be brought on by thoughts which are almost entirely imaginary, meaning that they are the furthest 'separated' from the life and death situations which brought 'acute stress' to our ancestors. However, even the often-imaginary stress of modern living, up to and including that which results from pressing deadlines at work, wreak havoc with your body. Stress is perhaps most damaging to the heart, especially if it is already vulnerable. Let's remember that stress can hamper the quality of an even highly comfortable life. Past age 50, what good is high-quality furniture or quiet neighbors when you're suffering from symptoms of acute stress such as:

(1) Cranky, forgetful or 'out of control' feelings. It doesn't take a rocket scientist to know that feeling 'stressed' can affect your ability to navigate your day. Even if your 'rational' brain disagrees (that is, even if you're not being chased by a wild animal), if you're so stressed that you feel edgy or 'out of control', make no mistake: your body thinks it is under attack. There are both immediate and long-term costs for these feelings. First, stress causes a hormone called cortisol to be released into the bloodstream and brain. Along with a range of other chemical processes, cortisol triggers feelings of tension, often of a sort which can override other brain functions (like rational problem solving). This leads to the sensation of being 'out of control.' In addition to such feelings being obviously dangerous (as in, who wants to worry about 'flying off the handle' due to some circumstance?), they can also cause severe consequences for the heart: Remember that hormone cortisol? Well, like most hormones, it is manufactured in the pancreas and released in response to stress. Unfortunately, just because cortisol was produced within the body, doesn't mean that it's good for you.

Prolonged exposure to the stresses of modern living is a circumstance for which your body can be said to have been 'unprepared': When modern people face stressors that are abstract and emotional, they face greater exposure to stress that our ancestors would have felt as life threatening, and thus risk a greater exposure to unhealthy 'cortisol flooding'. Additionally, the consequences of such 'flooding' are especially acute when they are considered in terms of heart health. A 2015 study from Maduka and colleagues found that over 200 'apparently healthy' young college students were so stressed by end-of-year exams, that blood testing performed before and after the exam period showed "a significant increase in serum cortisol" in the subjects – which was to be expected – but the blood testing also showed significant increases in serum (or 'overall') levels of adrenaline, as well as higher levels of both HDL and LDL cholesterol. The short version is that acute stress can damage the cardiac system, even when such stress is experienced over a relatively short period of time. Stress is a life-saving mechanism, meaning that people weren't ever intended to 'use' it so often.

(2) Reduced resilience/capacity to maintain homeostasis. The effect of stress on the body goes even deeper than the long-term consequences of continual 'cortisol flooding.' Instead, stress can affect the body's ability to regulate itself; acute stress can result in the disruption of the body's functional homeostatic equilibrium, or the body's dynamic equilibrium in continual adjustment to its environment. Homeostasis results from positive and negative feedback systems that trigger other systems or are themselves triggered in response to environmental stimuli. Like 'individual' body systems out of which homeostasis is contained (which manage temperature control, blood glucose levels, the oxygen cycle or osmoregulation [the control of water and salt concentrations in the body], etc.), homeostatic equilibrium is maintained without conscious thought. However, these many beneficial or critical feedback loops can be disrupted either individually or all at once in response to severe or unexpected environmental conditions. The most immediate and pressing consequence of homeostatic dysregulation is a reduction in resiliency, or your reduced ability to recover from illness and by extension, a reduced ability to adapt to your environment.

The human body is made up of dynamic systems, 'nested' in other dynamic systems, and they usually work as intended. The dynamic response that the body exercises in order to achieve homeostasis is known as 'allostasis.' A range of studies have shown that continual exposure to 'unusual' stressors (especially experienced over the long-term) can result in long-term disruption to both overall resiliency and to allostatic potential. The result of reduced resiliency can fall along a multiple vectors, all of which intertwine with heart health: One example can be seen in the ability the heart to properly respond to bodily and environmental factors: When allostatic resiliency is high, your blood pressure will rise when you go out for a light jog, causing some strain on the heart to achieve greater aerobic efficiency during the jog. Then your blood pressure goes back down again once you get back home and sit down on the couch. Simple.

However, when stress disrupts the body's allostatic potential and thus disrupts its overall resiliency, it can mean that blood pressure which goes up after a jog (or stressful experience) doesn't come down in a timely manner. Such consequences can be known as 'allostatic overload', and describe when the body's adaptation to stress doesn't 'shut off', or begins to do more harm than good. High blood pressure results in more stress, as well as damage to the heart. But this is only one example: Because homeostasis is also achieved across the neuroendocrine, autonomic, nervous, and immune systems, stress which impacts any of those systems can also cause damage the heart. This means that the potential heart consequences of stress are too many to list here, and can essentially 'travel' along any vulnerable systemic pathway the body has to offer.

(3) Additional examples of the heart consequences of stress include: Hypothalamic-pituitary-adrenal axis (HPA) dysregulation. The HPA axis is an important part of the body's overall stress response, and disrupting its ability to uphold equilibrium has been linked to the same predictors of reduced heart health as other dysregulation. Stress can also result in reduced energy and poor sleep. Reduced energy metabolism caused by stress is linked to hormonal and glucose factors. Worse than merely affecting quality of sleep (both actual and perceived), reduced waking energy levels from stress can weaken cardiac energy metabolism, meaning the energy system that keeps your heart running smoothly. Additionally, high and chronic stress can cause inflammation, leading to higher blood pressure and reducing serum levels of 'good' HDL cholesterol (which helps remove 'bad' artery-clogging LDL cholesterol from the bloodstream).

High stress has also been linked to anxiety, major depression and cognitive impairment as well as overall declines in health. In addition to causing higher serum adrenaline and cholesterol, stress (and the 'cortisol flooding' it causes) has been linked to other negative heart outcomes. These include higher levels of triglycerides (the blood lipids that can collect and harden in the arteries) and high blood sugar. Increased incidence of hyperglycemia causes increased diabetes risk, with diabetes itself posing a significant risk to heart health: The coronary implications of diabetes are much the same as the threat that diabetes poses to all the tissues of the body; runaway blood sugar threatens physical damage to the vessels and nerves of the heart.

When acute, 'out of control' incidents of stress occur dozens or hundreds of times in a lifetime, their damaging effects can compound upon the heart. It's no mystery why stress makes you cranky. But feeling out of control or unable to carefully consider the problems coming your way is only the 'surface' result of acute or high levels of stress. Below the surface and especially in the heart, stress can be deadly.

BUT IS THERE A REMEDY?

Now that we've plumbed the depths, how about some good news? Is there a proven remedy for stress? Well, the answer may not surprise you, but sort of.

We've already considered paths to reducing stress, and some of them seem to make very good sense: reducing stress can be achieved through exercise such as yoga, but also personal and spiritual practices like the giving of thanks, meditation or prayer, or even by deep breathing. Additionally, we've touched upon how stress can be reduced through pleasurable activities such as being in nature, interacting with pets, or through the protection of personal and professional boundaries. However, these factors represent only a 'surface'-level understanding of stress, in that these recommendations tend to reflect 'common wisdom' and not the results of discrete experimentation.

Perceived Stress. A good place to start is with the idea of perceived stress; the factor is given strong attention in a meta-review from Richardson and colleagues (2012), published in the American Journal of Cardiology. These researchers examined the role of 'perceived' stress in risk of heart attack and other adverse coronary event. In their study, they examined the links between the perception of stress and being afflicted by coronary heart disease. Across their assessment of six other studies with a combined 118,696 human subjects between them, Richardson and colleagues found that "high perceived stress is associated with a moderately increased risk of incident CHD." Put simply, we are shown here that perceived stress is just as relevant in day-to-day consciousness as stress which results from an actual, physical threat.

However, much like pain, the feeling of stress is subjective, meaning that it differs from person to person. It can be measured, however, under a host of scales with their readings reconciled with a range of conditions and characteristics for both the subject and environment. That said, perceived stress is an effective measure because people are generally good judges of their own stress levels; Cohen's (1994) Perceived Stress Scale emphasizes the importance of self-report, on the assumption that when it comes to adverse health conditions, people are unlikely to misrepresent themselves, especially if they might have something to gain by presenting their conditions 'as they are.' This is fortunate because it means that perceived stress can be considered 'actual' stress, and because any studies showing self-reported evidence of reduced stress might be cited as showing evidence of effective stress-reduction strategies.

Stress Best Practices. A good way to explore the 'best practices' of heart-healthy stress reduction is through examining how stress is controlled in 'high stress' fields and occupations. For instance, Rudaz and colleagues (2017) published a meta-review in the Journal of Contextual Behavioral Science concerning quantitative studies of mental health professionals' experience and views of mindfulness training, especially that which stresses acceptance of the self and others. Acceptance can be highly useful in reducing stress; in fact, the usefulness of training in the value of acceptance is so useful in reducing stress that it's part of the Serenity Prayer that one might hear recited in Alcoholics Anonymous or in other group support programs. Often credited to the Bible but actually written by the American theologian Reinbold Niebuhr (1892-1971), the prayer goes, "grant me the serenity to accept the things I cannot change / the courage to change the things I can / and wisdom to know the difference"). Put simply, stress can often result from an inability to 'let go', or from the irrational tendency to 'wallow' in bad feelings which result from stress. Mindfulness and acceptance training (which is achieved through mindfulness exercise) has been shown to prevent unnecessary stress in mental health professionals. Moreover, mindfulness/acceptance training was useful in preventing burnout among therapists, psychiatrists, and other professionals who work with high-needs people. Aggregated across dozens of studies, mindfulness-based interventions targeting mental health professionals were shown to have a moderate effect on perceived stress levels, as measured by self-report. Efficacy in these subjects (whose exposure to emotional stress is higher than the population as a whole) was interpreted as additional indication of the efficacy of this method.

Similarly, Guo et al. (2019) published a study in the journal Psychiatry Research showing that mindfulness-based stress reduction to be effective in reducing stress levels among pilot recruits in the military, a population for whom expectations are high, as well as levels of stress in the recruits. When explored in tandem with evidence from Rudaz et al. (2017), the concept of psychological resiliency comes up more than once. The idea is also raised by Fraess-Phillips and colleagues (2017) for the International Journal of Emergency Services, who found that mindfulness and self-acceptance training were effective in reducing levels of stress among firefighters. Interestingly, mindfulness and self-acceptance were found effective in reducing job-related stress even among firefighters who were afflicted by post-traumatic stress disorder, a factor which suggests its usefulness for military personnel. Unsurprisingly, PTSD is linked to poor heart health. In addition to mindfulness (being aware of one's surroundings, sensations, and environment), nursing research has also found effective stress-reduction in coping and adaptation methods, and by belief in an internal locus of control – that is, to believe that you are the 'captain of your own ship' – along with creating achievable goals and maintaining a positive mood. When combined with the strong evidence of mindfulness effectiveness and the ideas of acceptance, asserting that sort of 'control' can be said to 'fill out' a robust psychological defense against stress.

It follows that strategies found to be effective in reducing stress among those occupations for whom 'resting stress' is higher (psychiatric, military, emergency services, and medical personnel), may be the most effective in reducing stress in other communities as well. That is, if these strategies are good enough for younger people in jobs where they are under a great deal of stress, then they're likely good enough for the 50+ person who is only under a moderate level of stress.

Unfortunately, it appears that the downside of stress as a phenomenon measured through self-report is that interventions which purport to show an effective stress mitigation strategy, can be called into doubt due to environmental and situational factors alone. This perceptual factor means that when it comes to something as subjective as stress, there is no 'best solution.' Ultimately, stress is a personal journey of sorts, with few 'tried and true' methods to reduce its effect, except as a matter of personal choice. Earlier in life, you might have been able to 'skate by', so to speak, in a life with too much stress. One can imagine the young new parent, up all night with the baby and drinking coffee before dashing off to work on little to no sleep. But the resiliency of youth is far higher than that experienced past age 50, and the first, most vulnerable victim of reduced resiliency when you're under acute stress, is the heart.

Overview. Stress is a physical thing, and it causes physical damage to the heart, resulting from 'cortisol flooding' due to modern stressors that the body naturally, instinctively interprets as threats to your very survival. Over a long time, stress causes continual damage to the heart directly, and also by damaging the delicate systems that keep the body in equilibrium. 'Best practices' for stress reduction can be taken from stressful occupations, with military personnel, first responders, and psychiatric workers all finding strong reductions in self-reported stress after mindfulness training, especially that which emphasizes self-acceptance and acceptance of the environment and others, but also asserts the self as the 'locus' of control and the importance of achievable goals.

Let's take care of your heart, shall we?

REFERENCES

Cohen, S., Kamarck, T., & Mermelstein, R. (1994). Perceived stress scale. Measuring stress: A guide for health and social scientists, 10(2), 1-2.

Fraess-Phillips, A., Wagner, S., & Harris, R. L. (2017). Firefighters and traumatic stress: A review. International Journal of Emergency Services, 6(1), 67-80.

Guo, D., Sun, L., Yu, X., Liu, T., Wu, L., Sun, Z., ... & Liu, W. (2019). Mindfulness-based stress reduction improves the general health and stress of Chinese military recruits: A pilot study. Psychiatry Research, 281, 112571.

Lopaschuk, G. D., Karwi, Q. G., Tian, R., Wende, A. R., & Abel, E. D. (2021). Cardiac energy metabolism in heart failure. Circulation research, 128(10), 1487-1513.

Maduka, I. C., Neboh, E. E., & Ufelle, S. A. (2015). The relationship between serum cortisol, adrenaline, blood glucose and lipid profile of undergraduate students under examination stress. African health sciences, 15(1), 131-136.

Niebuhr, R. (1943). The serenity prayer. Bulletin of the Federal Council of Churches.

Richardson, S., Shaffer, J. A., Falzon, L., Krupka, D., Davidson, K. W., & Edmondson, D. (2012). Meta-analysis of perceived stress and its association with incident coronary heart disease. The American journal of cardiology, 110(12), 1711-1716.

Rudaz, M., Twohig, M. P., Ong, C. W., & Levin, M. E. (2017). Mindfulness and acceptance-based trainings for fostering self-care and reducing stress in mental health professionals: A systematic review. Journal of Contextual Behavioral Science, 6(4), 380-390.

♥

CHAPTER 8

THE GOALS OF HEART HEALTH, AND ACHIEVING FULFILLMENT

NOW THAT WE HAVE ESTABLISHED that stress is a physical thing and linked to poor heart health, it is time to explore the purpose of stress reduction (or indeed, any other recommendation made so far) in the context of heart health past age 50.

You might think this an odd choice, but when you peel back the layers of the onion, as it were, we come to recognize how it's a fool's errand to pursue heart health behaviors when the goal is only to prolong life. In actuality, to work toward this goal ("I must live as long as I can") is both to doom yourself to failure – we shan't dwell upon the fact and inevitability of death here – and to sabotage your long-term chances of strong health and longevity. But you may ask: If not to prolong life, what is the purpose of maintaining one's heart health? Why should I, for example, commit to reducing stress through acceptance and mindfulness, if not to live as long as I can?

Bear with me here: First, don't get discouraged. It's acceptable (even preferable) to motivate behaviors of exercise, healthy eating, or stress reduction, or any of the heart health recommendations we've covered so far, from a place of 'self-evident' purpose. That is, it's acceptable to view these as tasks to be performed without moment-to-moment awareness of their 'why.' However, it's inappropriate to use the goal of longevity alone to motivate those heart-healthy behaviors. This is unrealistic, and unlikely to pay long-term dividends. Sure, we'd all like to live forever, but there's a major difference between a life which was lengthy and one which was well-lived. And unfortunately, even a long life which is stressful places strain upon the heart.

With their first-place life expectancy of 85 years, the people of Japan live (on average) about 7 years longer than Americans. But even among the Japanese, studies have shown that stress and other adverse factors are just as strongly linked to poor heart health, and to higher age-adjusted risk of mortality, as they are in the U.S. No one would suggest that the Japanese don't live long lives. Yet studies like Suzuki et al. (2020) and Munakata (2018) show that the perhaps uniquely healthy people of Japan are just as susceptible to the ravages of stress (especially in overwork), or inactivity and even poor diet which results in adverse cardiovascular outcomes and general poor heart health. The point of this aside to the Far East is to stress that longevity alone is not a firm foundation upon which to rest your heart health motivation.

Why not? Well, heart health behavioral motivation is about quality of life, but heart health behaviors past age 50 can be hard work. The active, often-daily monitoring that these behaviors can require are often onerous. So too is heart health medication adherence and other maintenance or attention actions. These can become ever more tedious to manage, and with it, you're less likely to keep at them. Not for me, you might say. Perhaps that's true, but let's consider the impact of inappropriate motivation on long-term health behaviors, and your chances of heart healthy behavioral adherence.

Let's say that you logically recognize the value in taking your medication (and enduring medication side effects) for the purpose of not getting a stroke or heart attack. Simple enough, but let's also say you're only taking these medicines to prolong your life.

Over time and especially past age 50, the mere fact of your continuing to live (which, let's recall, was your sole motivation in the first place) may appear increasingly onerous or burdensome. The same can be said of other heart-healthy behaviors, such as abstaining from red meat or otherwise enduring the perceived self-denial of the heart-healthy diet. Finally, the path from sedentary lifestyle and into untrained 'beginner' exercise, even of a low-impact variety, can be rife with pain and discomfort.

Past chapters have shown that the criticality of such actions to heart health is not in doubt, but absent appropriate motivation, your enthusiasm can become increasingly lacking, leading to poor behavioral adherence. Why? It's simple: If you take on beneficial heart health behaviors with the goal of longevity alone, the negative aspects of the behaviors can come to dominate your frame of mind. In time, improper motivation means that you'll likely come to fixate upon how these behaviors are impeding upon your quality of life, regardless of the extent to which you know them to be beneficial. This means there's less of a chance that you'll keep them going. What use is it to live a long life, you may ask, if I must force myself to exercise, or to deprive myself of the foods I love, or take medication where the only outcome appears to be misery?

See how quickly a solitary motivator like 'longevity' falls apart? This failing is based in psychology, and how we tend to be poor judges of what is best for us.

Unfortunately, people tend to "overreact to perceived negative events — like passing on dessert — and underestimate our coping skills" (Shelly, 2022). This means that we can be blinded by the short-term negative consequences of heart-healthy behavior, leading to a greater likelihood of abandoning these behaviors altogether. This can result in your living for pleasure, or 'for today'. We can all recall someone who has adopted this attitude, but it's important to remember that such a person is often (or invariably) threatening their heart health. I'm not here to debate the morality of personal choice, only to show that heart health requires a body (and mind) which is committed not merely to life in the abstract, but to life in which you have so much to live for that the little difficulties and withholdings of heart health don't seem like such a high price to pay. I've found that when longevity outcomes are achieved in the face of threats to heart health, long life is less the result of tenacious adherence to heart-healthy behaviors – though these are necessary – as a 'byproduct' of a life which is well-lived, even happy.

You cannot pursue long life directly.

Instead, you can only 'trick' yourself into long life, through living a life in which the day-to-day benefits are so strong that heart healthy behaviors are a minor annoyance, or are even incorporated into the overall landscape of one's own healthy self-fulfillment.

This second idea informs the ideas to follow: In essence, the best way to motivate heart healthy behaviors is to incorporate them into your life in a way that you find personally satisfying and fulfilling. The last chapter touched on ways that you can reduce stress through direct and deliberate action, and focused on how stress is often the product of distinct (and achievable) thought patterns like mindfulness. However, this is not the 'end all' of stress reduction, nor does stress reduction precisely translate into good heart health past age 50. However, it is part of motivating heart health, along with comprehensive physical activity and the optimization of mental health, especially psychological fulfillment, all of which are vital ('stress-adjacent') factors that represent hardy foundations for a heart-healthy lifestyle, and in essence, the secret to long life.

No, really. I know it sounds glib, but let's take physical exercise as an example. We've already covered how exercise helps to strengthen muscles and endurance, but the benefits of daily exercise bear repeating. Exercise is a beneficial and low-cost heart health strategy fully customizable to specific needs with brief training, which helps to enhance balance, prevent falls, promote psychophysical well-being, and strengthen the muscles, including the vital muscle that is the heart. These facts are not in dispute! Along with mitigating the negative consequences of inactivity and sedentary lifestyle, regular low-to-moderate intensity physical activity (where there is elevated heart rate) is a critical aspect of heart health. Best of all, exercise helps enhance awareness of the body, leading to a greater likelihood of identifying potential health problems before they become deadly. So it follows that everyone would exercise, right?

It's more complicated than that: See, even if they fully understand the concrete benefits of regular physical exercise, people will still have trouble motivating such activity past age 50. See, the flawed idea of heart healthy action which is motivated by longevity alone, is that the cold logic of longevity can be easily thwarted by the emotions which result from immediate, short-term discomfort. Because we are predisposed to imbue short-term consequences with more gravity than long-term benefits, motivation to commit to a heart-healthy behavior can easily falter. As covered, this results in a lesser likelihood of adhering to a good plan after suffering initial negative consequences

However, studies like that by Herbert and colleagues (2022) or Di Lorito (2021) show that people with a positive wellbeing are more likely to adhere to a physical exercise regime. The same goes for other heart-healthy behaviors. So how do we give heart-healthy behaviors a fighting chance?

BY OPTIMIZING MENTAL HEALTH

Mental Health Past Age 50. Make no mistake: Mental health problems are not the province of the young, and if people today seem to succumb to these problems in greater numbers, it is only because awareness of mental health issues is now far stronger than it used to be. A commonly-cited statistic is that one in five adults past age 50 suffers from some sort of mental or neurological disorder, with dementia, depression, and substance abuse the most common among them (CDC, 2021).

Worse yet, people older than age 50 will often 'suffer in silence,' meaning that they are either unaware of the mental health condition they're suffering, they're not receiving appropriate treatment, or both. Now, it's probably not a mystery as to why these figures are relevant to heart health: Depression is implicated in suicide, but it can also "adversely affect the course and [complicate] the treatment of other chronic diseases," and thus it can complicate heart-related health maintenance behaviors, or long-term or postoperative cardiac outcomes (CDC, 2021). Depression can also complicate adherence to optimal long-term heart health behaviors. Treatment in old age focuses upon psychotropic medications such as selective serotonin reuptake inhibitors (SSRIs) or similar, typically aligned with talk therapy or other method of intentional mental health upkeep behaviors. The goals of talk therapy can be aligned with the stress reduction behaviors considered in the last chapter, especially ideas of forgiveness and acceptance, but such goals and outcomes are as varied as people are. In addition, alcohol abuse and other substance abuse behaviors are often unreported in individuals over 50, resulting in a greater likelihood of negative physical consequences, not to mention the socio-emotional toll taken by substance abuse behaviors at any age.

Dementia is perhaps the most tragic of these three; Unlike depression and even substance abuse behaviors, the individual with dementia can have a great deal of difficulty even recognizing that they are having a mental health problem, and as a result are largely (or even completely) dependent upon their caregivers for support. This isn't necessarily the 'end of the road' as far as mental health is concerned, but studies have associated improperly managed dementia with poorer heart health outcomes (Muqtadar et al., 2012), as well as 'vice versa', meaning that poorer heart health leads to increased risk of dementia (Stephan et al., 2017).

This second threat must not be underestimated: It has been shown that poor heart health results in "neurodegeneration" resulting from excessive "amyloid deposition", which results from abnormal antibodies (amyloids) accumulating in the heart and cardiovascular system, of which the body cannot dispose (Ow & Dunstan, 2014). Cardiac amyloidosis (also known as 'stiff heart syndrome') can result in arrhythmias and other complications, and has been associated with greater risk of general dementia as well as Alzheimer's disease (Ziskin et al., 2015).

Let's review: Mental or neurological disorders can complicate adherence to 'best practices' heart health recommendations. If you're depressed or afflicted by a substance abuse disorder, you have lower chances are of keeping to an exercise routine or heart-healthy diet, and lesser likelihood of avoiding or compensating for stress (aside from using maladaptive behaviors which may exacerbate heart health risk). Access to beneficial social and emotional resources (even inside the family) is also much-reduced past age 50, leading mental health problems with cardiac complications going untreated or even unrecognized as problems at all. So be careful! Poor mental health can have significant 'downstream' complications in terms of poor heart health, and poor heart health can result in poor mental health outcomes. However, researchers Levine and colleagues (2021) describe how there is currently a "preponderance of data [to] suggest that interventions to improve psychological health can have a beneficial impact on cardiovascular health," meaning this relationship works both ways (Levine et al., 2021). While the cardiac risk of excessive stress is the most acute psychological threat to heart health (Stephan et al., 2017), recent evidence has begun to associate long-term poor mental health – particularly depression – with the increased threat of cardiac illness, perhaps working along the same amyloid paths as dementia, or simply resulting from insufficient attention paid to health maintenance.

So – aside from medication, counseling and emotional supports (or other specific strategies) are there 'broader' paths to reducing mental health risk past age 50?

Yes! There are! And as with the 'goal' of heart health in the first place, this extraordinary strategy for optimizing mental health centers upon the idea of fulfillment.

Psychological Outcomes and Fulfillment. Previous sections have considered how it is foolish to focus upon maintaining heart health for the sake of long life alone. But if not long life for its own sake, what is the purpose of long life? Answers to this question may seem self-evident, but let's consider what the science has to say about optimizing psychological outcomes past age 50.

First, the good news. Recent studies have shown considerable advancement in the treatment of chronic diseases of age, particularly those of the heart. This has resulted in an extension of "disability-free life expectancy", leading to a "longevity dividend", during which those older than age 50 can now appreciate far-stronger benefits of "better education, [and] more flexible age norms related to family formation, work and retirement," as well as "greater financial security, and…opportunities to be involved in their communities", than was available in the past (Diehl et al., 2020). Put simply, medicine and society today are 'friendlier' to people over age 50, and people in this group now appreciate a greater chance to achieve psychological fulfillment which is directly linked to superior heart outcomes (Levine et al., 2021).

But what is psychological fulfillment? Simple. Psychological fulfillment is subjective wellbeing as a more or less 'permanent' condition, meaning that you know it when you feel it. Fortunately, people over age 50 tend to report higher subjective wellbeing than middle-aged people, with acutely reduced worry and stress past age 60 (Steptoe et al., 2015). This suggests that the same factors which have resulted in the 'longevity dividend' have resulted in greater happiness and fulfillment in those past age 50. We'll get into the 'why' of this phenomenon in a second, but let's first reiterate that lack of psychological wellbeing is a matter of subjective perception. This means that if you're not sure you're experiencing a state of wellbeing, then you probably aren't.

But what are the paths to wellbeing, and by extension, toward fulfillment, from which great heart health benefits can be appreciated? Again, while these may seem self-evident, let's review the science of this matter: In short, subjective wellbeing hinges upon positive subjective estimates of different aspects of life, including "physical and mental health, financial position, [existence of] social supports and connectedness to community, opportunities for growth and ability to achieve their goals," as well as a "general sense of purpose and satisfaction with [one's] life course" (Levine et al., 2021).

How can these be achieved? Unfortunately, life circumstances may interfere with the ability to optimize your financial position, opportunities for growth or ability to achieve your goals (though the American audience to whom this work is addressed may have an easier time achieving these goals with their related heart health benefits, than those in more repressive nations). This means that many psychological factors which result in strong heart health are a matter of chance. However, environmental, economic, and other circumstantial factors aside, the most important path to psychological wellbeing is through emphasizing healthy relationships, especially in family, and by fostering healthy connections with one's community. People are social animals, and much of psychological fulfillment results from being useful and beneficial to one's family, friends, and wider peer group. A notable theory known as socioemotional selectivity theory suggests that as people grow older, they "accumulate emotional wisdom that leads to selection of more emotionally satisfying events, friendships, and experiences", and that this increased ability to seek out positive social experiences results in the 'disproportionate' level of wellbeing reported among people older than age 50 (Steptoe et al., 2021). If there's one major 'takeaway' from this chapter, it's to work on your relationships, both at home and in the world, for they are precious.

But what if you've always had trouble making and keeping friends?

Well, fulfillment can also result from focusing on yourself. Really, fulfillment represents the ability to 'follow' whatever paths result from subjective wellbeing, and subjective wellbeing is wherever you can find it, but especially in family and community. When it comes to the self, subjective wellbeing results from focus on maintaining one's own individual identity and life path, or from 'adhering' to one's expectations or beliefs about what a 'good life' should be. If you're struggling in this regard, just imagine what might make your 10-year-old self the happiest, and if that's not feasible, remember the dreams of your early adulthood. Fulfillment can result from virtually anything, so long as you're true to your own desires: You can lead a life of pure asceticism and give your every cent and hour of time to your community, and still not be as fulfilled as someone who recognizes pleasure as their major priority, and works to pursue that goal alone. That said, the predilection of people over age 50 to find fulfillment in community (especially through caregiver or volunteer work) means that you might find more success if you follow a selfless path, but the point is be true to yourself.

It's all about averages: Truth to your identity means a greater likelihood of subjective wellbeing, which causes a greater likelihood of fulfillment. This leads to a greater likelihood that you'll adhere to heart-healthy behaviors, resulting in a greater statistical likelihood of good heart health. Put simply, happiness leads to heart health.

Cheers!

REFERENCES

Centers for Disease Control and Prevention (2021). The State of Mental Health and Aging in America. Retrieved from ttps://www.cdc.gov/aging/pdf/mental_health.pdf

Diehl, M., Smyer, M. A., & Mehrotra, C. M. (2020). Optimizing aging: A call for a new narrative. American Psychologist, 75(4), 577.

Di Lorito, C., Long, A., Byrne, A., Harwood, R. H., Gladman, J. R., Schneider, S., ... & van der Wardt, V. (2021). Exercise interventions for older adults: A systematic review of meta-analyses. Journal of Sport and Health Science, 10(1), 29-47.

Herbert, C., Meixner, F., Wiebking, C., & Gilg, V. (2020). Regular physical activity, short-term exercise, mental health, and well-being among university students: the results of an online and a laboratory study. Frontiers in psychology, 11, 509.

Levine, G. N., Cohen, B. E., Commodore-Mensah, Y., et al. (2021). Psychological health, well-being, and the mind-heart-body connection: a scientific statement from the American Heart Association. Circulation, 143(10), e763-e783.

Ow, S. Y., & Dunstan, D. E. (2014). A brief overview of amyloids and Alzheimer's disease. Protein Science, 23(10), 1315-1331.

Muqtadar, H., Testai, F. D., & Gorelick, P. B. (2012). The dementia of cardiac disease. Current cardiology reports, 14(6), 732-740.

Stephan, B., Harrison, S. L., Keage, H. A., Babateen, A., Robinson, L., & Siervo, M. (2017). Cardiovascular disease, the nitric oxide pathway and risk of cognitive impairment and dementia. Current cardiology reports, 19(9), 1-8.

Steptoe, A., Deaton, A., & Stone, A. A. (2015). Psychological wellbeing, health and ageing. Lancet, 385(9968), 640.

Suzuki, Y., Maeda, N., Hirado, D., Shirakawa, T., & Urabe, Y. (2020). Physical activity changes and its risk factors among community-dwelling Japanese older adults during the COVID-19 epidemic: Associations with subjective well-being and health-related quality of life. International journal of environmental research and public health, 17(18), 6591.

Munakata, M. (2018). Clinical significance of stress-related increase in blood pressure: \ current evidence in office and out-of-office settings. Hypertension research, 41(8), 553-569.

Ziskin, J. L., Greicius, M. D., Zhu, W., Okumu, A. N., Adams, C. M., & Plowey, E. D. (2015). Neuropathologic analysis of Tyr69His TTR variant meningovascular amyloidosis with dementia. Acta neuropathologica communications, 3(1), 1-7.

CHAPTER 9

♥

FINANCIAL STABILITY AND ACHIEVING 'PEACE OF MIND' PAST AGE 50

WHO CAN IGNORE THE PROBLEMS of the present day? It seems that everywhere we go, we are confronted with messaging and news that is troublesome, or gets under your skin. Maybe it was always this way, but the increasing pace of the modern world means that there are more opportunities than ever to come across news and current events that are upsetting. You probably know where I'm going with this. To come across a bit of information which causes you to feel angry or unsettled, even if this information is not directly related to your life, it is nonetheless the same thing as stress which results from unwelcome events or tragic developments more localized to your own life.

It has been shown that prolonged exposure to bad news, especially that which is emotionally arousing, can be just as damaging to your long-term heart health as more localized stressors, especially past the age of 50 (Davis, 2019). So what kind of news leads to stress? On one hand, news about what's going on in the world, either nearby or far away, can cause emotional stress and thus contribute to unnecessary stressors which imperil heart health. That said, it's not always easy to discern between the news stories that are likely to cause you unnecessary or unhealthy levels of grief or difficulty, from those which are necessary to understanding the world around you. So what's the solution? As with many things in life, the answer appears to be moderation.

In more than one study, it has been found that the consumption of bad news is not a problem in of itself, but rather, news consumption only becomes a problem and a dangerous source of stress when it is compulsive, meaning that such news consumption takes up parts of your day that you would rather spend focusing on your own life. It can certainly feel good to be well informed, but it's important to not get 'carried away', as it were (Boukes & Vliegenthart, 2017; Oppenheimer et al., 2011).

But what about bad news that you can't ignore, or erect meaningful barriers and boundaries to protect yourself against? One major example of such unavoidable bad news can come in the form of bad financial news. Say you lose your job, or the index fund in which your retirement is invested takes a nose dive, or any one of a galaxy of factors comes into play which causes you to feel financially insecure. This is a tremendous stressor, but unlike many others, solutions are not immediately apparent. Where do you go from there? Let's explore the links between financial security and achieving the low levels of stress most conducive to good heart health.

Recall that stress outcomes which are negative for heart health result in a 'fight-or-flight' response, and in the release of stress hormones adrenaline and cortisol. Although it may seem strange, the same is true of stress reactions to bad news, even bad news which is financial in nature. It is not necessarily difficult to recognize why. Financial insecurity can mean fear and a great deal of concern about the road ahead, and one's ability to survive and thrive moving forward. Especially as one passes the age of 50, and can no longer rely upon their physical body as much as they once did, financial security may be all that is keeping your fragile sense of self intact.

Negative financial security can result in negative mental health outcomes, particularly anxiety and depression, but it can also manifest as increased levels of constant, day-to-day stress. This puts an extraordinary burden upon the heart, and can lead to reduced quality of life. Additionally, it may go without saying, but bears repeating here: heart health requires a constant and active relationship with one's care providers, meaning that financial and security can result in reduced heart health as a function of reduced ability to access care. This means that financial insecurity can worsen health.

No matter what, it is an unfortunate reality that financial security can purchase quality care, not merely when it comes to the health of the heart, but with a range of other health outcomes. To this end, the best means by which deleterious stress damaging to heart health can be prevented, is through maintaining financial security sufficient to ensure that one is able to afford not merely reactionary care – such as care received after a heart attack or other damaging event – but proactive, preventive care as well (Thayer et al., 2012). By extension, it may become necessary to maintain one's productive potential and ability to earn money past age 50, in order to put oneself in the best possible position to obtain necessary care before suffering a stroke or heart attack.

That said, this work does recognize that financial stability and security is often difficult to come by, and that not everyone is able to achieve such a state on their own.

This is where maintaining strong and supportive relationships comes into play, the importance of which cannot be stressed past age 50. Your family and friends are lifelines during potential times of financial insecurity or deprivation. Although this is not necessarily true in every case, through maintaining strong relationships with family and friends, you certainly put yourself in a stronger position to 'throw yourself on their mercy', so to speak, should you face overwhelming financial difficulty. Not only will they be likely to provide you with the security that you require, but the ability to ask friends or family for help in times of need (even if such needs never arise) will help reduce stress that you may experience as a result of financial insecurity. It's all related!

But is it possible to pull yourself out of financial insecurity? Unfortunately, past the age of 50, it is often more difficult to work, especially if you're used to working long hours at physically demanding jobs. That said, it may be necessary to find new work to shore up your financial security, perhaps seasonal work or some other temporary arrangement. You may be lucky enough to have a pension, or to draw from Social Security, but make no mistake: you must take care of your financial situation, both for the sake of your welfare and those around you, as well as to reduce the stress that you experience as a result of having an uncertain financial standing.

Debt, in particular, that major aspect of financial insecurity, has been linked to high stress and by extension, worse heart health outcomes (Kuruvilla & Jacob, 2007). It is in debt where the link between bad news and heart unhealthy outcomes is found: Suboptimal financial choices lead to debt, but it falls upon debt collectors to receive just repayment. If you are not in a position to repay those debts, then the simple act of checking the mail can become a source of tremendous stress, as well as answering the telephone. Even though we are only talking about numbers in a ledger, the link between stress and negative heart health manifests in this situation as well. It is best to ensure that your debts are repaid, and that you are not being hounded by debt collectors, as that state of affairs is known to be linked to poor heart health (Kuruvilla & Jacob, 2007). I'm sure you can picture it: no matter how hard you try to keep your blood pressure low and reduce damaging stress, you cannot control who calls or sends notices to your house. All you can do is try to ensure that you are in as strong a financial position as possible. This can require diligence and thrift, but mostly paying strong attention to your interpersonal relationships. Moreover, maintaining financial security might require the kind of humility and pragmatism that might allow you to take a job that you might not have found dignified in years past. Unfortunately, your heart doesn't much care how you earn the money you need to stave off deprivation or debt collectors. All your heart cares about is that you are not under threat. If you haven't considered it this way before, please do so now: financial insecurity represents a direct threat to your heart health, and unfortunately, it is critical that you figure out a way – anyway – to put your financial house in order past the age of 50.

This can take the form caregiving work for friends and family, or seasonal or retail work, or even non-physically demanding telework if you can perform it (Goughler & Trunzo, 2005). You might even be able to rely upon friends and family, however much this might appear a 'last resort' solution in the face of financial difficulty. The long and short of it is that you cannot neglect your financial stability, as to do so risks incurring stressors for which you may be unprepared, and which can cause heart trouble.

But what is the purpose of financial security? Like past questions raised in this volume, such as that considering the purpose of heart health, the answer might seem self-evident, but this is not necessarily the case. You work towards financial security in order to provide for yourself and others, and to ensure that unexpected problems or difficulties are only that, difficulties, and not truly catastrophic or deadly. The goal of financial security is to be able to hold your head high and to recognize that the world around you cannot cause you such terrible financial hardship. More precisely, financial security is a path to peace of mind. Peace of mind is something you've no doubt heard of before, but it bears repeating. Peace of mind is the absence of worry or anxiety, or as close to it as you may be capable of achieving. Particularly in America, peace of mind often goes hand in hand with financial security, but it is also the end result of a range of other recommendations that have been made throughout this work. Past age 50, it is not merely a matter of one's life being more pleasurable and satisfying than a life consumed by anxiety and doubt. Instead, peace of mind can mean superior heart health as well (Al-Shabiani et al., 2015). But how can this be achieved?

It is all a matter of optimizing your life outcomes.

How can this be accomplished? It's simple! An optimal state of affairs past age 50 is to have a life which is free of scarcity and deprivation, with a healthy diet and lots of exercise, and in which you experience 'personal fulfillment.' Not coincidentally, these factors are linked to long-term heart health, with the idea of "successful aging" also often tied to personal resolve and the continuance of physical activity (Rozanova, 2010). By extension, it is best to approach personal fulfillment from an idea of successful aging, typically and best in a manner which is personalized to you. This means going to the doctor. It's from here that we consider the idea of healthcare participation.

Healthcare participation is more than just answering questions and obeying orders. Instead, it's a relationship, one in which your health depends on your open and honest involvement in your own care practice. Make no question: An optimal life past age 50 is one where you are strongly invested in your own care, responsible and professional at appointments, and diligent in following your doctor's advice.

But you must do no more than that!

What does this mean? Well, let's talk about what is not meant by healthcare participation. All too often nowadays people are content to do their 'own research', especially when it comes to online exploration of health options and opportunities, or just seeking out health information and advice online. No question, that kind of activity can feel like proper and appropriate healthcare participation, because in many ways, it is designed to appear that way. Moreover, the choice to do one's own research when it comes to health and wellness can even seem to 'fit in' alongside other actions intended to secure you financially. What use is financial security, you might say, when it comes to reducing my heart-unhealthy stress, if I must pay through the nose consulting with my doctor over every little thing? After all, you're a smart cookie! Why should you bother your general practitioner or worse yet, a specialist, wasting both their time and your money getting information you could have gotten for free, not to mention faster and more conveniently online? And lastly, if peace of mind is your ultimate goal, then why shouldn't you get the information you need, right now?

Why not indeed! After all, the internet has been a monumental boon to the sharing and exchange of information; no longer do we need to go to a physical library or bookstore to read up about heart health. Better yet, we are freed to describe our every symptom into the text bar of a search engine, and draw upon the wisdom of the ages, available right at our fingertips. And all of this is, to some extent, true.

The problem is that the internet is also a tremendously untrustworthy source of what is often but not always accurate information. First, let's reiterate; the internet (or the first page of search engine results) is no replacement for direct advice from a physician or practitioner. What the internet is, is convenient, and perennially 'on hand' to seemingly address every concern and anxiety we have. However, worse than simply not speaking to a doctor, the internet can be a source of dangerous misinformation, or more frequently, the source of information which – while accurate – may be designed to upset you. Let me be clear: Heart health information online is rarely inaccurate, not exactly. But it is important to remain skeptical and cautious of the often emotional or compulsive experience of obtaining information online. A significant stress potential and heart threat exists there which must not be overlooked.

Let's say that you have chest symptoms and rather than visiting your cardiologist or heart specialist, you use WebMD, the well-known commercial website. Now, the draw of websites like WebMD is that they are free, and readily provide extensive information about any medical or health topic the user requests. And they are reliable, an important quality nowadays. After all, we're living through a golden age of information, but also an epidemic of misinformation, and your wellbeing may depend upon your ability to distinguish between the two (Krishna & Thompson, 2019). So let's say fear of misinformation is the reason you went to WebMD in the first place; after all, you don't want unnecessary worry, so why not use the 'brand name' in health information?

So you go on WebMD and pop in the symptoms you can describe, and before you know it, you've gone down an internet 'rabbit hole', clicking link after link and reading page after page until hours have gone by, and you discover, much to your dismay, that you have no more peace of mind than before you started.

What happened?

It's simple: For the people at WebMD to reach enough page-views to sell enough ads to be profitable against their network costs, they need you to spend as much time on WebMD as possible. Oddly, you might have emerged from hours on WebMD, still anxious but proud of yourself when it was done, as if you had studied for a difficult test.

But don't be mistaken: 'Binging' internet health content and advice is also no replacement for actual care and personalized advice, and it may even make things worse. So really, what happened? Sadly, it was like this: WebMD and thousands of websites and internet services like it uses subtle tricks of writing and design and markup to keep you interested and moving about within their 'ecosystem', and you got hooked. It's nothing to be ashamed of, and it's very common these days (Lin et al., 2019).

When it comes down to it, WebMD and other sites like it (especially social media) don't especially care why you spent hours on their site, just that you did. So while the information they provide might not be inaccurate, it is not necessarily the best information for you to consume if you are looking to keep your stress at a heart-healthy level. Social media and many commercial sites recognize that user 'engagement' is motivated by "entertainment, information seeking, personal utility and convenience", but the line between the first two – entertainment and information-seeking – can get very blurry, especially when it comes to maladaptive behaviors in web users (Al-Menayes, 2015). For instance, nothing can stop you from reading WebMD while afraid for your heart health, nor from intentionally exposing yourself to upsetting information because you're convinced that 'the only way out is through' and that reading article after article is how you take control of your own medical stewardship. What WebMD or other health sites do, is capitalize on that anxiety, and generously allow you to choose to anxiously gorge yourself on health information, so long as you continue to do so on their site.

That doesn't sound like me, you might say. I wouldn't allow that to happen. That's wonderful! But you mustn't let down your guard. Even as an adjunct to proper medical advice – say, as a means of understanding advice and orders and prescriptions duly given by your provider – health information obtained online is not especially useful. Not if you're looking to avoid unnecessary sources of stress, that is. Look at it this way: Is it rational to use a service, however convenient, where health information and advice is depersonalized and designed to be as entertaining as possible, even if the entertainment value it provides can also make your concerns worse or your fears grow?

No? Then instead I implore you: Go to your doctor or practitioner. Take the time and build a relationship with these caregivers, and ask them questions and listen to their advice. And for crying out loud,

Don't Do Your Own Research!

Unless you're an expert, the internet is a minefield of misinformation right now, and a lot of information sources are designed to be addictive. But even if the internet was a pristine library, ideal in every way, there's the matter of how researching heart health is not your responsibility! We live in a complex society, and my role is that of a heart doctor. Please allow me and my colleagues to fulfill our roles and please, I implore you, trust that our advice is correct. After all, the research is the hard part (when done properly, it takes years!); your only responsibility is to follow best practices.

Let's review. It is important to attend closely to your financial stability because financial instability can contribute to significant heart unhealthy stress factors. However, this is accomplished, the key goal of financial stability is to ensure peace of mind. Peace of mind is the absence of significant stressors, and is in many ways the secret to heart health past age 50. Importantly, a core aspect of heart health past age 50 is healthcare participation. This means building and maintaining a strong relationship with your caregiver, but also trusting what they have to say and not presuming to know more than they do. Beware bad news, and the temptation to use the internet as a replacement for seeking medical advice. It is important to surrender oneself to the understanding that you cannot become an expert in a field overnight, simply because your interest in it is strong. In fact, you may upset yourself further, leading to stress which worsens the heart condition you're investigating. Instead, allow centuries of scientific development to 'carry' your burden and trust your provider. This way you can limit another source of stress linked to poor heart health, and lessen a source of unnecessary responsibility.

Take it easy!

WORKS CITED

Al-Menayes, J. J. (2015). Motivations for using social media: An exploratory factor analysis. International Journal of Psychological Studies, 7(1), 43.

Boukes, M., & Vliegenthart, R. (2017). News consumption and its unpleasant side effect: Studying the effect of hard and soft news exposure on mental well-being over time. Journal of Media Psychology: Theories, Methods, and Applications, 29(3), 137.

Davis, A. (2019). How our emotions affect our heart health. Retrieved from https://www.eehealth.org/blog/2019/03/emotions-heart-health/

Krishna, A., & Thompson, T. L. (2021). Misinformation about health: a review of health communication and misinformation scholarship. American behavioral scientist, 65(2), 316-332.

Lim, M. S., & Choi, S. B. (2017). Stress caused by social media network applications and user responses. Multimedia Tools and Applications, 76(17), 17685-17698.

Lin, W. S., Chen, H. R., Lee, T. S. H., & Feng, J. Y. (2019). Role of social anxiety on high engagement and addictive behavior in the context of social networking sites. Data Technologies and Applications, 53(2), 156-170.

Oppenheimer, S., Villa, Y., & Apter, A. (2011). Effects of prolonged exposure to terrorism on Israeli youth: Stress-related responses as a function of place of residence, news consumption, and gender. Adolescent Psychiatry, 1(2), 152-162.

Rozanova, J. (2010). Discourse of successful aging in The Globe & Mail: Insights from critical gerontology. Journal of aging studies, 24(4), 213-222.

Thayer, J. F., Åhs, F., Fredrikson, M., Sollers III, J. J., & Wager, T. D. (2012). A meta-analysis of heart rate variability and neuroimaging studies: implications for heart rate variability as a marker of stress and health. Neuroscience & Bio behavioral Reviews, 36(2), 747-756.

CHAPTER 10

♥

OVERVIEW AND POINTS OF SPECIAL EMPHASIS

So WHERE DOES THIS LEAVE us? Near the end of the book, that is for sure! The present exploration of health past age 50 has hopefully produced in the dutiful reader a newfound appreciation for the importance of the heart, and with it a finer recognition of the systems that can aid in optimizing heart health past middle age. How to end such an exploration? My idea was this: Throughout this work, I have occasionally found reason to seize the attention of the reader through the use of bold text, or declarative text,

Like this!

And it is for that reason that this concluding chapter begins by reiterating the points that necessitated such energetic use of emphasis. Following this 'walk down memory lane,' as it were, it also offers an overview of other salient points and specific recommendations, if they were not already discussed, particularly by extending the discussion of independent medical research begun in Chapter 9. In total, this chapter shows why it is important to remember to care for the heart actively and consciously, indeed, we must show the heart the respect and diligence it shows us in return, and strive for heart health past age 50 that is motivated not by fear but instead by a duty to 'match' the heart's everlasting power with our own discipline and habitual consistency.

POINTS OF SPECIAL EMPHASIS

In Chapter 1, The Multiple Paths to Long and Healthy Life, special emphasis was placed on how health outlooks are best when considered a global concept, albeit one in which heart health assumes a deservedly heavy importance. That said, we must remember that all systems of the body, along with behavior, outlook, and psychology, count toward happiness and long life potential, not just those with which we are typically or actively aware. While it may be tempting to neglect heart health or physical health in general to focus on a life 'of the mind', mental health remains but one system among many. This means that while you may imagine that your very existence 'exists' within or flows through the 'seat' of consciousness in the mind (that is, in the brain), psychological fulfillment is also situated in other systems of the body, even those about which the conscious mind is not typically aware.

One such system is situated in the heart. Heart health reflects its own or global health in silence, meaning the heart does not 'announce itself' to the consciousness except if there is reason to 'sound the alarm', like by palpitations or chest pain. Sadly, the lack of 'low-level' monitoring potential in the heart (as might forewarn the conscious mind of plaque accumulating on the arteries) is a deficiency of the body for which only the use of 'best practices' in preventive heart healthcare, represent the optimal solution.

In Chapter 2, Health throughout the Life Cycle, strong emphasis was placed on the adaptive trait known as resiliency, meaning your capacity to overcome challenges and to maintain health and function despite loss, disability, or disease. It is essential that resiliency be a focus of your heart health journey, due to the heart damage that can result from stress.

Resiliency behaviors have been linked to better 'peace of mind' past age 50. Interestingly, 'getting' to resiliency behaviors (that produce peace of mind and slow the resting heart rate) might be easier than adopting specific heart-healthy behaviors. It's true! It is more likely that you will ultimately attend to your heart health if your life is worth living, meaning if you are inattentive to your heart health today, you may have a 'happiness' or a 'fulfillment' problem, rather than a heart problem per se. Resiliency exists in the pursuit of passions and interests, and through connection with family, and through the pursuit of strong purpose in life, and in my view, the best form of purpose in life is in personally-meaningful activity that incorporates physical exercise. Such outcomes as central to wellbeing are explored in Chapter 9.

In Chapter 3, Preventive Care Overview, special attention was paid to the things that are most likely to kill you, and what are not. Statistically, violent crime will not kill you, nor will terrorism, nor natural disasters. Heck, even if you're in a disaster-prone region on the morning of a disaster, you're unlikely to be killed in a natural disaster. Things that will kill you are stroke, heart disease, and cancer. Also automobile accidents, but that's a story for another day. Because it always bears repeating, here we go: Quit smoking, look both ways when you cross the street, and pay attention to your heart health. Every other bit of medical advice must be informed by a healthy and active relationship with your healthcare provider. Meaning you must never be a slouch when it comes to making appointments and attending t your preventive care! Remain current with all vaccinations, including against COVID-19 but also influenza, and discuss different health maintenance behaviors and medications with your primary care provider. Undergo proper breast cancer or colorectal cancer screenings at the appropriate age, when such screenings are appropriate. But above all, reduce sedentary lifestyle, quit smoking, and adopt a global 'life and longevity' mindset.

In Chapter 4, The Preventive Care Mindset' and Heart Health Over the Lifespan, a special emphasis was placed on why diets tend to fail. It was then boldly declared that no diet could fail if the changes in dietary intake were motivated by a view of preventive care which emphasized 'long-term thinking' of a special sort. This transitioned into a recommendation to diet (or engage in all heart-healthy behavior) motivated by a view of the needs of the self, far into the future. 'Future-orientation' is very important, because it provides an easy shorthand for recognizing the necessity of limited but concerted, daily, conscious action to optimize heart health through your present activity.

Inattention to a future perspective is described as unwise, and as more likely to indicate your succumbing to the 'sunk cost' fallacy – throwing 'good' money after 'bad' – with your health. An example of this is by through continuing to adhere to heart-unhealthy behaviors because of the strain or discomfort that adoption of new behaviors is expected to cause. However, one must 'rip the Band-Aid off' with heart health, as it were, and the path to courage and strength in this regard is to not 'fixate' on the downside, meaning dwelling on the idea of what you are losing today. Instead, you work for the benefit of the future body that you will inhabit one day, and for your loved ones of today and tomorrow. Additionally, longevity is useless if quality of life is low.

In Chapter 5, Modifiable Risk Factors for Atherosclerosis and Other Heart Disease, heart anatomy and physiology was covered, along with the specific risk factors for disease of the heart to which we are all exposed. Special emphasis was given for the value and even criticality of physical exercise, and the limitations imposed by the sedentary lifestyle. Although cardiovascular science may have taken some well-deserved jeers some years back after the publication of reports declaring that based upon new evidence, 'sitting is the new smoking' (Heart Foundation, 2019), the fact remains that people were not meant to sit. Rather, the best way to optimize your heart health is by leading the kind of physical existence that your earliest ancestor might understand, at least to the greatest extent that you can. This does not mean abandoning the comforts of modern society to live far from civilization, but it does mean engaging in vigorous cardiovascular exercise with some regularity. The secret to exercise is that your body needs to feel that it is necessary. This means you have to get your heart rate up habitually enough that your body learns that the exercise is necessary for survival. After 3-6 months, this results in 'feedback' gains for heart health, after the heart – jewel that it is – grows stronger and more efficient, to match your new activity level (even past age 50!). Just because we live in a society that allows a couch bound, sedentary existence, does not mean that we should partake, especially when your heart health is on the line.

In Chapter 6, Optimizing Heart Health Past Age 50 the key take-away concerned medication adherence. So once again: Take your meds. Especially statins. Statins have been a miracle for heart health that have saved tens of thousands of lives. But they cause uncomfortable side effects, and are associated with higher blood glucose and can be comorbid in type-2 diabetes. Enter into a medication regimen with the full cooperation of your physician, after reconciling your past experience with medication against the potential discomfort of side effects. Don't change your dosage without speaking to a doctor, don't avoid discussing side effects that are affecting your usage, especially if they cause discomfort. Recognize that the side effects of medication can be difficult but the alternative is progressive heart disease or dysfunction, and that especially once you've already had a heart attack or stroke, daily medication for life may be necessary. This is an uncomfortable truth, but poor medication adherence means increased risk of suffering further adverse heart events, or death. Just take your meds. To lighten matters somewhat, Chapter 6 returned to place additional emphasis on the importance of exercise and healthful eating, and presented a number of foods known to reduce inflammation associated with cardiovascular disease.

Chapter 7, Mental Health and Stress and Heart Health in Old Age, strongly emphasized the importance of limiting stress. Stress or moments of strain lead to the release of cortisol, which means that the body thinks that it is under attack. However, body systems involving 'cortisol flooding' during a 'fight or flight' moment are unprepared for the stressors of the modern world. Constant, low-level stress can result in an increase in serum cortisol, meaning that whenever you're under enough stress that your blood starts pumping, your body thinks that it is under attack. The result of such continual, low-level 'cortisol flooding' is that (in addition to crankiness and sleep troubles) your body develops a reduced ability to maintain homeostasis, and is more susceptible to heart disease.

Reduce your stress. Damage to homeostasis resulting from high stress can even adversely affect cardiac energy metabolism, or the heart's energy system, along with causing artery-clogging inflammation, leading to high blood pressure and reduced serum ('good') HDL cholesterol. Please take the time to assess your own stress levels and determine how your stress can be reduced. Mindfulness and acceptance training (like the "serenity" prayer) may be useful, along with pursuing a life with an internal locus of control. Ultimately, stress is a personal journey through what is best remembered as a physical phenomenon with physical consequences for the heart.

In Chapter 8, The Goals of Heart Health, and Achieving Fulfillment, this work returned to the suggestion from Chapter 2, and the idea that there are two options when it comes to heart health: The first is heart health motivated for its 'own sake', in order to extend life because it is 'best' to live for as long as one is able. The other is heart health as a 'consequence' of a life lived with purpose. Truthfully, I would imagine that many readers have not reflected on 'why' they wish to love a long life, aside from the wish to provide for their loved ones. Even that selfless wish feeds into the idea of life lived for as long as possible and for its 'own sake', a posture that neglects both how habits are formed and how the heart responds to different environmental factors. Follow all of the explicit health advice in this book, but remember the why of heart health.

It's like this: Even the most attentive heart-healthy individual can find it difficult to cope with medication side effects, or they may truly 'feel the pain' of a heart-healthy diet. Unfortunately, if you're fixating on side effects and discomforts, it may be because you are pursuing heart health not out of desire but obligation. Most importantly, heart health is at its easiest when there is mental health (including talk therapy and medication), and strong mental health may aid in the adoption of physical habits that are most conducive to global heart health outcomes. What are these goals? They can be anything, so long as they involve physical activity and improve the health of the heart.

In Chapter 9, Financial Stability and Achieving 'Peace of Mind' Past Age 50, we discussed bad news, which can often seem to follow us around, especially in the current 'supercharged' media landscape. Unsurprisingly, bad news is just as bad for the heart as (for instance) workplace stress, in that it represents another source of urgent threat that cannot be immediately rectified, thus suggesting the 'cortisol flooding' linked to stress-induced heart illness. Turn off the news. Once that's done, make sure that you do not have any significant financial strain in your life. This may be the most important goal of your life, but you must work until you complete this goal because financial stress is deadly. Debt, in particular, has been implicated for the pain and damage that it can cause the heart, when considered in terms of the 'cortisol flooding' suffered in response to a debt notice. Other chapters have emphasized the value of agency in one's life, and the way that debt inhibits agency has been linked to strain which, once again, is damaging to heart health. Unfortunately, the best solution here is to simply get your finances in order, by whatever means possible, if only for the heart health benefits.

Finally, Chapter 9 ended by announcing a new rule for heart health: Do not do your own research. I hope that the tone it set did not seem presumptuous, nor was it intended to spread a message of ignorance. Instead, this was a defense of pre-internet information specialization, at least when it comes to matters of one's own likelihood of being afflicted by a given disorder. But here, once again: I would not object to proliferation of exploitative platforms like WebMD if the whole country had a college-level understanding of statistics and probability, and even a high school understanding of medical examination or anatomy. But since we don't, we may neglect our health for years, only to develop symptoms and rush to the 'open arms' of WebMD. 'Binging' negative health data or anxiously perusing medical databases elevates our sense of health danger, as well as our sense of personal risk when obscure viruses and conditions happen to match our current symptoms. So, once again: Things that will kill you are stroke, heart disease, and cancer. And car accidents. Quit smoking and pay attention to your heart health, look both ways, and talk to your doctor.

We are essentially incapable of evaluating our own health in a dispassionate manner, and it is the doctor's actual job to provide accurate diagnoses, along with advice and orders designed to save and prolong our lives. Most of all, medicine is a useful service, while untrained use of medical research databases can exacerbate stress or worsen heart illness. Above all, come to embrace the idea of 'surrendering' authority to a physician in health matters: This may appear to run counter to heart health's often-focus upon the importance of personal agency and the internal locus of control, but trust me on this one:

You can afford to take a back-seat to the doctor when it comes to heart health. Not because you cannot identify symptoms or read a website, but because to fixate upon accumulating knowledge is often to express one's intent to 'discover' a hidden secret (whether in the form of an obscure condition or treatment), like searching for hidden treasure. The unfortunate truth is that life with heart disease can often mean a lot of discomfort, and no amount of amateur medical research is going to lead to outcomes or recommendations that do not reflect the prevailing heart health wisdom. Statistically, we are most likely are not unique, so it is wisest to abandon the ego and just keep to best practices, by approaching heart health from a perspective of what is most likely to harm your heart.

The 'boring' truth that we may not wish to admit, and the 'pull' of WebMD and other sites offering the contrary, is that smoking, sedentary lifestyle, stress, and medication no adherence are at the core of what harms heart health. But so what if it's boring? Let's be boring together! Past 50, we've earned the right to slow down a little. So please, stay away from these websites and do not do your own research. Instead focus on life change and new, heart-healthy goals.

IN CONCLUSION, your heart has carried you since before you were born; it is the precious clock that runs your body, and a biological miracle worthy of our respect. Also worthy of our respect is the self who does not yet exist, that 'future' self who will either enjoy or painfully endure the body that we provide them. By ignoring the future, we insult the heart. What is best is to 'circumvent' the heart, by giving it, essentially, 'something to do.' Modern society allows us to lead sedentary lifestyles but they cause the heart to grow weak and clogged with plaque. Even under the limited physical expectations of modern society, you must engage in enough physical exercise to 'trick' the heart into thinking that regular exercise is a survival necessity. Your path to this outcome is your own responsibility. But this a very sustainable path to adopting the physical exercise regimen most useful to heart heath. Healthful eating and stress reduction are useful, as is medication adherence, but if you want to live to be 90, you can benefit most from getting the heart to work 'for you', by strengthening it through regular cardiovascular exercise – and this is critical here – exercise which you enjoy. Only you know what that means, but be creative! How did you exercise and play as a child? Follow your joy (and all safety recommendations), but find joy in exercise.

Most of all, don't think of any of these recommendations in terms of what they will remove from your life, except for unhealthy or unwise habits and behaviors. Instead, strive to develop pleasurable habits which 'coincide' with heart health (like personally-enjoyable exercise). Best of all, strive to develop exercise habits that might be enjoyed by some 'future' you. I think that you might agree, they will thank you for it.

REFERENCE

Heart Foundation (2019). Is Sitting The New Smoking? Retrieved from https://theheartfoundation.org/2019/08/10/is-sitting-the-new-smoking/

Printed in the United States
by Baker & Taylor Publisher Services